# Multicultural Perspectives in Communication Disorders

# Multicultural Perspectives in Communication Disorders

**Robert Martin Screen, Ph.D.**
Hampton University
Hampton, Virginia

**Noma Bennett Anderson, Ph.D.**
Howard University
Washington, D.C.

**SINGULAR PUBLISHING GROUP, INC.**
San Diego, California

**Singular Publishing Group, Inc.**
4284 41st Street
San Diego, California 92105-1197

© 1994 by Singular Publishing Group, Inc.

Typeset in 10/12 Andover by House Graphics
Printed in the United States of America by McNaughton & Gunn

All rights, including that of translation, reserved. No part of this publication may be reproduced, stored in a retrieval system, or transmitted in any form or by any means, electronic, mechanical, recording, or otherwise, without the prior written permission of the publisher.

**Library of Congress Cataloging-in-Publication Data**

Screen, Robert Martin.
    Multicultural perspectives in communication disorders / Robert Martin Screen, Noma B. Anderson.
        p.    cm.
    Includes bibliographical references and index.
    ISBN 1-56593-265-X
    1. Communication disorders—Cross-cultural studies.
2. Intercultural communication.    I. Anderson, Noma B.    II. Title.
RC429.S39   1994
616.85′5—dc20
                                                                                             93-49681
                                                                                               CIP

# Contents

Foreword by Diane Scott, Director — vii
Office of Multicultural Affairs
American Speech-Language-Hearing Association

Preface — ix

Acknowledgments — xi

Chapter 1  **An Understanding of the Professions** — 1

Chapter 2  **Multicultural Participation in the Professions of Audiology and Speech-Language Pathology** — 17

Chapter 3  **The ASHA and Cultural Diversity** — 25

Chapter 4  **The Black Caucus of the American Speech and Hearing Association: A History** — 31
By M. Eugene Wiggins
University of the District of Columbia

Chapter 5  **Beyond the Black Caucus: The National Black Association for Speech Language and Hearing, the Native American Caucus of the ASHA, and the Hispanic Caucus of the ASHA** — 43

Chapter 6  **Legal and Ethical Issues in Communication Disorders Affecting Multicultural Populations** — 51

Chapter 7  **Language Development in an Ethnolinguistically Diverse Population: Speakers of Black English Vernacular** — 65

Chapter 8  **Counseling Minorities in Communication Disorders** — 81

Chapter 9  **Communication Disorders Among Multicultural Populations** — 95

Chapter 10  **Profiles of Audiologists and Speech-Language Pathologists Representing Diverse Cultural and Linguistic Groups** — 109

References — 117

Index — 123

# Foreword

Cultural and linguistic diversity is changing the face of America today. Based on the 1990 census, African Americans, Hispanic Americans, Asian Americans, and American Indians comprise a quarter of the U.S. population. Moreover, these nonwhite populations are growing faster than the white population. If current birth rates and immigration patterns continue, people of color will comprise nearly one third of the U.S. population by the year 2010 and almost half by the year 2050.

The reality of cultural and linguistic diversity must, therefore, be addressed by the professions of speech-language pathology and audiology. Cultural and linguistic diversity have critical implications not only for children and adults in need of speech, language, and hearing services, but for students trained to work with these individuals. Faculty and students need to understand the impact of culture and language on communication development, communication patterns, and communication disorders.

In January 1992 a group of American Speech-Language-Hearing Association (ASHA) members who had previously attended an ASHA-sponsored Institute on Teaching Cultural Diversity developed a document entitled *Multicultural Professional Education Program—Administered Audit* to help education programs monitor their progress toward cultural diversity within the curriculum. Among the methods mentioned for increasing cultural diversity was the use of textbooks that adequately cover multicultural information. This introductory textbook is, therefore, both timely and significant. This book provides a multicultural perspective for students as they first begin their studies in communication sciences and disorders. The authors cover not only communication disorders within multicultural populations but also discuss cultural diversity within the professions themselves. The culturally and linguistically diverse speech-language pathologists and audiologists profiled in the book can offer immediate role models for students from the same or even different backgrounds.

An added bonus of this book is that exposing students to a multicultural perspective early in their studies can lead to their continued examination of the disciplines of audiology and speech-language pathology from that perspective. They may then be better prepared to confront the untold number of culturally related professional issues they will inevitably face as this century ends and the twenty-first century begins.

Diane M. Scott<br>
Director, Office of Multicultural Affairs<br>
American Speech-Language-Hearing Association

# Preface

As we approach a new century and the year 2000, we are becoming increasingly aware of the changing demographics in our society regarding ethnicity. In other words, there will be a significant increase in multiculturalism in our society characterized by marked differences in age, ethnicity, and racial composition of our population.

The implications of these changing demographics upon the professions of speech, language, and hearing should be significant. At the present time in our professions, the majority of the personnel are European American, and they are essentially monolingual speakers of English. As we project toward the future, however, it is predicted that approximately one third of school-age children will be either African American, Asian American, or Hispanic American, and these children will be speakers of English as well as dialects and languages other than English.

Additional research on our emerging population for the year 2000 has revealed that there are at least six states with an African American, Hispanic, Asian, and Native American public school enrollment of at least 35% or more, and another 12 states in which these students make up 34-35% of the enrollment (Ramirez, 1988). Even as of this writing, there are some cities in the United States whereby students of color comprise a majority of the school population. For example, current figures released by the state of Texas reveal that better than 51% of kindergarten children are Hispanic. The children of color enrolled in school programs in cities such as Miami, Philadelphia, and Baltimore are 71, 73, and 80%, respectively. In essence, if these trends continue, it is possible that by the year 2000, one out of every three students across the United States will be African American, Asian, or Hispanic. As we relate these figures to the professions of speech, language, and hearing, it becomes apparent that the caseload for the future will be comprised of minority students. Are we ready to met the needs of this changing society?

The purpose of this text is to be of assistance in this regard. Specifically, this text is designed to provide students and others with information about multiculturalism and the involvement of the American Speech-Language-Hearing Association (ASHA) and multicultural speech, language and hearing organizations in the development of this new interest. We feel that students and professionals alike must learn and know as much as possible about multicultural issues in communication sciences and disorders. There are so many areas of multiculturalism that need to be researched and examined further. There need to be more textbooks on this subject, more clinical approaches that address multiculturalism, and more professionals who are socioculturally aware as they practice the professions of speech, language, and hearing. The ASHA has conducted a number of endeavors to expand the multicultural curricular offerings of graduate programs. The ASHA's Office of Multicultural Affairs has sponsored a series of Professional Education Conferences where faculty from graduate communication sciences and disorders gathered to be taught by faculty who are experts in cultural and linguistic diversity. They were also given extensive resource literature for the purpose of incorporating this much-needed information into programs' curriculum.

As we look to the future, multiculturalism presents some issues that our professions will have to give serious attention. For example, where are we now with foreign language requirements in our universities? After 1980, many schools began dropping their foreign language requirements for the bachelor's degree, and departments of foreign language across the nation began to suffer because of dwindling enrollments. Fortunately this trend is changing because there are tremendous needs for bilingual speech-language pathologists and audiologists. Another challenge for our professions is the need for speech-language pathologists to join diagnostic and educational/intervention teams along with teachers of English as a Second Language (ESL) and classroom teachers. Using a team approach, the educational and communication strengths and needs of children whose first language is a language other than English need to be addressed, and appropriate individualized and group programming needs be developed, all within the context of sociocultural awareness and respect. Speech-language pathologists and audiologists need to learn much more about the communication processes and needs of adult and elderly individuals from multicultural populations. Assessment and clinical programming would become much more effective, efficient, and competent if our professions were to expand their understanding of communication diversity across the human age span from a multicultural perspective.

# Acknowledgments

A text of this type, on a field still so new, must be the combined effort of a number of people in helping us to fulfill many roles.

Our first thanks must go to our graduate students who toiled endlessly in helping to put small pieces of information together from a multitude of sources. A special note of thanks in this regard goes to Janean Lawyea of Hampton University.

The professional assistance of M. Eugene Wiggins of the University of the District of Columbia and Susan F. Robinson of the District of Columbia Public Schools was a godsend. The information each of them provided on the history of the Black Caucus and NBASLH, respectively, has never been published, and we are certain it will be beneficial to all who need to put NBASLH into perspective. Similarly, we are grateful for the professional assistance of Barbara Nunnery of the University of Arizona and Alexandra Heinsen-Combs of Richmond Hill, New York, for providing such valuable information on the Native American Caucus and the Hispanic Caucus, respectively.

We would like to thank Dr. Diane Scott, newly appointed Director of the ASHA Office of Multicultural Affairs, for writing the Foreword to this text. We wish you good fortune in your position and promise you our constant support. We appreciate the assistance you provided as we were compiling information for this project.

We want to thank those professionals from our respective departments who formed a group of distinguished reviewers and supporters. Among those persons are Dr. Pollie Saunders Murphy, Dr. Donna R. Brooks, and Mrs. Felicia B. Johnson of Hampton University, and Dr. Orlando L. Taylor, Dr. Shelly Chabon, Dr. Dorian Lee-Wilkerson, Mrs. Lemmietta McNeilly, and Mr. Abe Tishman of Howard University. We would also like to thank Dr. Fay Vaughn-Cooke and Dr. Wilhelmina Wright-Harp, of the University of the District of Columbia, for their encouragement and assistance.

We are indebted to all of you for your significant contributions to this project.

# Dedication

This book is dedicated to all of our students at Hampton and Howard Universities and to the inspirational leadership we have received over the years from Lorraine Cole of the Office of Minority Concerns (renamed the Office of Multicultural Affairs in July 1993) of the American Speech-Language-Hearing Association. For Lorraine Cole, we hope that this text will be a token of the appreciation that we have for the inspiration and example you gave us in the area of multiculturalism. For our students, we are hopeful that this text will serve as a challenge to you as you prepare to become contributing professionals, remembering to reach back and help others.

# 1

# An Understanding of the Professions

As a student who is looking ahead to several years of study and learning about the disciplines of communication sciences and disorders, you may not, at this stage in your education, be too sure about what lies ahead. You probably are becoming bombarded with terms that may be rather vague, or maybe even confusing: *communication sciences and disorders, audiology, audiologist, speech-language pathology, speech-language pathologist, American Speech-Language-Hearing Association, ASHA, and NBASLH.* Family and friends may be asking you to tell them something about your major. When they ask you what is your major, and you respond "communication sciences and disorders," or "communication disorders," or "speech-language pathology and audiology," they, as well as you, may be unsure of this terminology. Audiology and speech-language pathology are professions about which many people are unaware.

As you embark on a major in communication sciences and disorders, we, the authors of this text, want to provide you with a unique introductory experience, and we wish to express our excitement about your academic and professional career decision. Over the past few years something exciting has begun to occur across the country—more and more people are discovering the professions of audiology and speech-language pathology, and more and more individuals are applying to undergraduate and graduate communication sciences and disorders programs. There are several reasons for the increased interest in speech-language pathology and in audiology. One reason is that there are severe shortages of audiologists and speech-language pathologists in schools, hospitals, rehabilitation centers, nursing homes, universities, home health care agencies, and child development centers.

A second reason is that audiology and speech-language pathology are such diverse fields that broad opportunities exist for those who work in these fields. Communication disorders specialists work in schools (45.7% of ASHA members*[1]), colleges and universities (7.5% of ASHA members*), health care facilities (38.8% of ASHA members*), and industrial facilities (0.4% ASHA members*). Most ASHA members provide direct services to individuals with communication disorders (73.7%*); many ASHA members are administrators (10.6%); many are college and university faculty (4.2%); many are special education teachers (4.1%); many are consultants (2.3%); and some are researchers (0.9%).

Audiologists and speech-language pathologists provide communication assessment and (re)habilitation services to persons across the entire life span, from infancy to old age. Audiologists and speech-language pathologists work with a diversity of individuals who have difficulty communicating. People with disorders of communication are young and old; rich and poor; female and male; from all ethnic groups; and live in cities, towns, suburbs, and rural areas. They are people who have suffered a stroke; people with disordered vocal quality; people having difficulty learning to correctly produce speech sounds; people with fluency difficulties; people with physical disabilities; people communicating via augmentative communication devices; infants who are born with developmental disabilities; people who have experienced traumatic brain injury; people with hearing loss; people with cerebral palsy; people with amplification or assistive listening devices; people with mental retardation; and school-age children who express themselves using immature grammar. Working with such a diversity of individuals and such a wide range of disabilities makes the professions of audiology and speech-language pathology ever changing and forever challenging. These professions constantly experience explosions of information and technology. Audiology and speech-language pathology are dynamic, always evolving, fields of practice.

A third reason for the increase in interest in the fields of audiology and speech-language pathology is that people are discovering that these are rewarding professions. Communication is an important human behavior that is essential for successful interpersonal relating, for career success, and for academic success. Without the skills and tools of effective and appropriate communication one's life lacks an impor-

---

[1]* *Demographic Profile of the ASHA Membership (April 1, 1993)*, prepared by ASHA Research Division

tant quality dimension. Audiologists and speech-language pathologists improve the quality of life for those who are experiencing communication disabilities. People who want to work in professions that "make a difference" select audiology and speech-language pathology.

The American Speech-Language-Hearing Association (ASHA) is the professional association of audiologists and speech-language pathologists. The ASHA provides guidelines for professional practice, awards certification to audiologists and speech-language pathologists, accredits educational programs and service delivery agencies, disseminates basic and applied research and service delivery information through its publications, supports the National Student Speech, Language and Hearing Association (NSSLHA), organizes special interest divisions to advance collaboration around specific areas of practice, lobbies state and federal governments to advance the professions of audiology and speech-language pathology, advocates for and educates consumers, holds scientific and technical conferences and meetings, and engages in myriad functions.

This chapter presents an overview of the roles and responsibilities of audiologists and speech-language pathologists. The chapter, and this entire text, stresses the professional challenges that are created as the fields of audiology and speech-language pathology respond to multiculturalism. One reason for framing an introductory text around the multicultural picture is because many persons from multicultural populations who present with communication disabilities have historically been underserved. By underserved we mean that persons who are in need of communication therapy do not receive therapy, or do not receive a full range of communication services. Also, in the May, 1992 issue of *ASHA*, Thomas Smith, director of the ASHA's information and member marketing services, wrote: "African Americans, Hispanics, and Asian Americans have little knowledge of communication disorders and even less knowledge of the professionals trained and certified to offer treatment for communication disorders" (p. 53). While this may not be a completely accurate statement, Mr. Smith's statement does highlight a dilemma within our professions. For people of color to be better served, it will be necessary to gather information and present it to students early in their educational careers.

## MULTICULTURAL PERSPECTIVES IN COMMUNICATION DISORDERS

Why is it important for there to be a textbook on this topic? There are essentially three answers to that question.

One, there has been too little attention paid to understanding communication development, communication patterns, and communication disorders among ethnolinguistically diverse populations. As the United States progresses into the next millennium, ethnic groups, long regarded as minority groups, will instead be constituents of a new majority. One predictor of this demographic shift is two contrasting trends occurring simultaneously in this country. Together both will change the complexions of our nation. One of these changes is the "browning of America." By that we mean that persons from nonwhite populations are increasing in number, via immigration and childbirth, while the white populations are experiencing close to zero population growth. In contrast, there is also the "graying of America," which speaks to the increased life span of Americans. The significant increase in life expectancy tends to be observed more among the white elderly than nonwhite populations. One result of these two population changes is that there is significant population growth at the youngest end of the life span, and this growth is occurring more among ethnolinguistically diverse populations, and, there is significant population growth at the oldest end of the life span, and this growth is occurring more among white populations.

The "browning of America" is creating professional challenges for a number of professions. For communication sciences and disorders, the increasing number of persons from ethnolinguistically diverse populations has made audiologists and speech-language pathologists unsure of many of the theoretical principles of communication and communication development as well as the clinical procedures that provide the foundation of these professions. Uncertainty arises about the effectiveness of traditional approaches. In fact, from a survey conducted in the late 1980s, 77% of speech-language pathologists indicated that they did not feel prepared to serve clients who are from culturally and linguistically diverse populations (Campbell, 1985).

The basis for this lack of preparation regarding ethnolinguistically diverse populations and communication is because, historically, research in communication sciences and disorders has been conducted using white, middle-class individuals as subjects. Very early on in your study of audiology and speech-language pathology, you will discover that these are two research-based professions. From the research on communication development and communication behaviors, norms or standards were gleaned which became the basis for the development of diagnostic procedures in our fields. The diagnostic assumptions, diagnostic instruments, and diagnostics norms of our fields are based on research. From the diagnostic principles come our intervention principles, assumptions, and procedures. Thus, our rehabilitation is based on research. Professionals have begun to question the extent to which one can assume that the traditional research that was conducted with monolingual and monocultural white subjects is generalizable to nonwhite individuals. If the research is not inclusive of diverse social-cultural-linguistic groups, then one must question the degree to which diagnostic and therapy principles are valid for individuals from ethnolinguistically diverse groups.

A significant effect of the lack of research with ethnolinguistically diverse individuals is the lack of appreciation of linguistic variation that existed prior to the 1970s. Orlando Taylor, 1992 recipient of the ASHA's Honors of the Association, writes "While I was a graduate assistant . . . in 1958–60, I worked with many clients who had foreign accents, which were considered at the time to be a disorder meriting clinical intervention. . . . This experience caused me to raise serious questions about negative labeling of English that was *normally* reflective of influences from another language. This practice became even more disturbing to me during the 1960s as the civil rights movement gripped the nation. Eventually, cultural considerations became important to our understanding of normal and pathological communication" (Chabon, Cole, Culatta, Lorendo, & Terry, 1990, p. 13).

Taylor is referring to the "civil rights movement" within our professions that exploded during the 1970s. One succinct phrase that has gained tremendous professional import is *language difference versus language disorder.* Prior to the social awakening within the fields of communication disorders, anyone who did not speak Standard American English (SAE) was labeled language disordered and became a candidate for language therapy. The research and writings of many speech-language pathologists and sociolinguists were focused on the study of normal communication patterns and behaviors among culturally and linguistically diverse (i.e., not white, middle-class) families. Their documentation of varieties of normal language as spoken by diverse populations led to greater understanding of language difference. Documentation of language differences is necessary so that the diagnosis of communication disorders can be based upon knowledge of the individual's own communication norms.

This research introduced sociolinguistic concepts and vocabulary to the field of speech-language pathology. The term *dialect* was understood as being a rule-governed variety of a language. Speech-language pathologists began to recognize that the *many* varieties of English spoken by the U.S. population are influenced by geography, ethnicity, age, sex, education, and profession. Speech-language pathologists learned that every child acquires the language forms spoken in his or her speech community. Speech-language pathologists learned that everyone speaks a dialect. Speech-language pathologists learned that no dialect is superior, or inferior, to any other dialect. Speech-language pathologists learned that the social esteem, or the lack of esteem, given to particular dialects is not because of any linguistic factors, but instead is related to the degree of social esteem, or the lack of esteem, the majority culture feels for the speakers of that dialect. Can you think of one example of a dialect that is held in high regard? Can you think of a dialect that is held in low regard? Can you relate its status to the speakers or to linguistic factors? Moreover, there is limited empirically based knowledge about the influence of second language learning on communication development.

Thus, given this lack of full understanding of dialects of American English, given the state of limited knowledge about second language development, consider the professional dilemma facing speech-language pathologists as they are called on to assess and treat the communication disorders of increasing numbers of immigrants speaking many languages other than English and persons whose dialects vary from SAE. So there is little doubt that 77% of speech-language pathologists feel poorly prepared to meet the clinical needs of persons who are culturally and linguistically different from traditional mainstream American culture (Campbell, 1985).

A second reason that this textbook is needed is because many persons with communication disorders who are from ethnolinguistically diverse populations and/or are economically disadvantaged are too often underserved by audiologists and speech-language pathologists. One reason for this may be that our professions have traditionally been quite monocultural in perspective and philosophy. For audiologists and speech-language pathologists to work effectively with individuals from diverse populations, they must gain an understanding and awareness of cultural diversity. Such sociocultural awareness is now federally mandated for those professionals who service persons from 0 through 21 years of age with communication disorders and families. Speech-language pathologists, audiologists, occupational therapists, physical therapists, social workers, nutritionists, nurses, service coordinators, and others must all work within the context of culturally competent, community-based, family centered service delivery. All professionals must strive for increased cultural sensitivity toward cultures different from their own.

As you advance and mature within these professions, it is important to recognize that language and communication are cultural. It would be impossible for speech-language pathologists to diagnose and treat communication disorders without doing so within a context of sociocultural awareness. As a speech-language pathologist or an audiologist it will be important for you to not have a monocultural perspective to normal and disordered communication. Federal legislation, P.L. 99-457, requires that individuals 0 through 21 years of age receive services that are provided in a socioculturally appropriate and sensitive perspective. As our professions strive toward sociocultural sensitivity, our professional services will be more accommodating to and accepted by those who are from nonmainstream cultural and linguistic groups.

Low-income persons are also a population that is underserved. The effect of low income and poverty on individuals with communication disorders and their families is severe. Poverty creates tremendous barriers: barriers to access to services, barriers to awareness of available resources, and barriers to the utilization of educational and health care systems. Many middle-class families readily seek the services of audiologists and speech-language pathologists; however, many low-income families do not.

Many individuals from these cultural groups, as well as from low-income families, utilize speech-language pathology and audiology services differently from how these services are utilized by white middle-class families. Many nonmainstream individuals do not utilize mainstream service delivery agencies early on because of mistrust and lack of finances.

The third reason for this textbook is there are too few persons of color in this field. Chapter 4, "Minority Participation in the Professions," discusses the small number of people of color who are members of the ASHA. April, 1993, demographic data from ASHA state that 6.1% of ASHA members are from ethnolinguistically diverse populations. Research data reveal that 2.5% of ASHA members are African Americans, 1.7% are Hispanics, 1.6% are Asian Americans or Pacific Islanders, and 0.3% are American Indians or Alaskan Natives. Audiology and speech-language pathology are exciting professions that can embrace all persons.

## MULTICULTURAL CHALLENGES

In 1989, Lorraine Cole, while Director of the ASHA Office of Minority Concerns (in July, 1993 this office was renamed the Office of Multicultural Affairs), wrote about multicultural challenges facing our professions (Cole, 1989). The remainder of this chapter will present and discuss views related to Cole's eight multicultural challenges.

**1. More Minorities with Communication Disorders.** Since there has been an increase in the number of immigrants from Third World countries and since there is greater population growth among families of color, there are more "minority" persons living in the United States than in past decades. The consequence of this change in the U.S. population is that more persons of color are identified as communicatively disabled than have been identified prior to these years of population shifts. We are not advancing the position that there is a greater proportion of communication disorders among persons of color than among European Americans. What this challenge refers to is that presently audiologists and speech-language pathologists are providing services to more ethnolinguistically diverse families than we have in the past. As mentioned earlier, communication services must be provided in a socioculturally appropriate context. One major deterrent to culturally competent service delivery has been that audiologists and speech-language pathologists have received little education from their undergraduate and graduate programs on cultural and linguistic diversity (Anderson & Lee-Wilkerson, 1993). The ASHA is addressing this omission. During the past several years, the ASHA has sponsored professional education conferences to provide information on cultural and linguistic diversity to faculty from communication sciences and disorders programs so they can incorporate this information into their curricula. The ASHA also addresses multiculturalism by requiring that master's programs provide academic and clinical experiences on cultural and linguistic diversity to their students to meet accreditation standards. This accreditation standard went into effect January 1993. All master's programs must now include coursework and clinical practicum experiences addressing multiculturalism.

**2. More Minority Children Born At-Risk.** The term at-risk refers to a child presenting with one or a number of conditions that are recognized as having the potential to cause developmental disabilities. Examples of at-risk conditions are prematurity, respiratory difficulties, chromosomal disorders, low birth weight, prenatal drug exposure, neurological immaturity, HIV-positive diagnosis, and cerebral palsy. Identification, assessment, and intervention services that are provided to at-risk children are referred to as early intervention services. Many speech-language pathologists and audiologists are employed in early identification and early intervention settings. Many of the children seen by facilities that provide early intervention services are from ethnolinguistically diverse populations. There are a number of reasons for the large numbers of children born at-risk. One, as discussed above, the number of families from ethnolinguistically diverse populations is increasing; therefore, more children from such families will be a part of the at-risk population. Two, a large number of children born to poor families are at-risk for developmental disabilities. The effects of low income and poverty can be significant because too often mothers of low-income families have inadequate prenatal care and poor maternal health. This places the unborn and the neonate at-risk for conditions such as prematurity, infant malnutrition, low birth weight, and growth retardation. Low birth weight infants are at-risk for conditions such as brain damage, cerebral palsy, mental retardation, and learning disabilities (Anderson & McNeilly, 1992).

3. **Different Etiologies and Prevalence.** The five basic categories of communication disorders are: disorders of articulation (difficulty producing the speech sounds of one's language); disorders of fluency (speech production characterized by sound, word and phrase repetitions, sound prolongations, vocal blocks, speech anxieties, etc., that call attention to themselves and interrupt the flow of communication); disorders of language (difficulty processing and comprehending communication and/or the delayed or deviant development of the ability to produce appropriate communication, based on the communication norms of one's language community); disorders of voice (difficulty producing and sustaining appropriate vocal quality; pitch and/or volume, given one's age, sex, and cultural environment); and disorders of hearing (the loss of one's ability to hear adequately for communication).

The term *etiology* refers to the cause of a disorder; *prevalence* refers to the number of existing cases of a particular disorder. For the most part, communication disorders have been studied in Euro-American populations, and little information exists regarding multicultural diversity in the etiologies and prevalences of communication disorders. Epidemiologic information of communication disorders has staggered entries in the literature spanning several decades. Some of the knowledge that is known about cultural diversity is:

a. Otitis media, inflammation and fluid within the middle ear, shows highest prevalence among American Indians, followed by Asians, followed by white Americans, followed by African Americans (Scott, in press).
b. Presbycusis, progressive hearing loss among the elderly due to the aging process, shows multicultural prevalence trends. African American women maintain their hearing thresholds the best over time, followed by European American women and African American men, followed by European American men (Royster, Driscoll, Thomas, & Royster, 1980).
c. Sickle cell anemia is a disorder that affects persons of African ancestry. Communication disorders, particularly hearing loss, have been associated with this disorder (Payne & Stockman, 1979; Scott, in press).
d. Low birth weight is a condition that is often associated with developmental delay. A high proportion of babies born with low birth weight are African American infants.

Recent research indicates that regardless of income, education, and prenatal care, more African American babies are born with low birth weights than infants from white families (Schoendorf, Hogue, Kleinman, & Rowley, 1992). Thus, a predisposition, or tendency, for lower birth weights may be a contributing factor in the high number of African American babies born at-risk for developmental delay.

e. High levels of lead in children's blood has been related to both communication disorders and to ethnicity. The communication disorder that is associated with high lead levels in the blood is delayed language comprehension. It appears that elevated levels of lead in the blood have been found to be related to pigmentation of the skin. Apparently, African American children present with high lead blood levels, followed by Hispanic children, followed by white children (Mayfield, 1984). High blood lead levels are associated with physical disorders and mental retardation.

f. Congenital HIV infection, human immunodeficiency virus, and AIDS, acquired immune deficiency syndrome, affect children from all cultural groups; however, the majority of the pediatric AIDS and HIV-positive cases are children of color. In 1991, the Public Health Service estimated that 3,200 children were diagnosed with AIDS and that approximately 10,000 to 20,000 were found to be HIV-positive. Of children under the age of 5 with a HIV-positive diagnosis, approximately 56% are African American and 26% are Hispanic (Anderson & McNeilly, 1992; Crocker & Cohen, 1990). Two disabilities that result from AIDS are mental retardation and encephaly. Both of these conditions are etiologies for delayed communication development.

**4. More Difficulty Establishing Norms.** The diagnosis of communication disorders is done principally through the use of testing. Some diagnostic tests have used African Americans and/or Hispanics within their standardization sample; however, most tests were developed by studying the communication behaviors of middle-class white Americans. The purpose of utilizing subjects for test standardization is that their communication behaviors become the basis for the development of the test norms from which test scores are derived. The problem with using a homogeneous standardization sample of subjects for the development of test norms is that, when individuals who are not members of that specific population are tested, the test norms are not as valid.

Attempts to evaluate a client's communication development using norms that are not representative of the client is referred to as biased assessment. The assessment is biased because the client is being judged by the norms from a population different from him or her. In the case of people of color, if the standardization norms are from a sample of only white subjects, then there is the great possibility that the client can be misdiagnosed. There is the possibility that a communication *difference* could be diagnosed incorrectly as a communication *disorder*.

Cole (1989) writes that there is more difficulty establishing norms for multicultural populations because of the tremendous social, ethnic, linguistic, and cultural diversity that exist among all people. If a test was normed on populations that included Spanish-speaking individuals, what linguistic norms are being used? For example, if the test was normed in Washington, D.C., and if Spanish-speaking persons were invited to participate in a norming study, most would be Spanish-speakers from Central America and Spanish-speakers from Puerto Rico. Many authorities in linguistics and in speech-language pathology would question the reasonableness of including two different Spanish-speaking groups. Then, would it be advisable for a speech-language pathologist in California to use this test and its norms to assess the communication development of Spanish-speaking clients in California? What if the client and her family immigrated from Mexico?

Imagine that you are a speech-language pathologist who is preparing for a diagnostic, and also imagine that you have at your disposal norms for various ethnic groups, and imagine that an African American child is your diagnostic client. Which norms would you use? Would you use your "African American norms" because this is an African American child? As stated earlier, there is tremendous social, ethnic, linguistic, and cultural diversity among all people. Would ethnicity be the sole factor you would use to select the test? Other cultural variables, such as social-economic background, parents' expectations, educational experiences, and communication style may make the use of the "African American norms" inappropriate. Taylor (in press) has stressed that race and culture are not synonymous.

Moreover, Vaughn-Cooke (1983) presents an important political statement that cautions us about the use of various test norms for several ethnic-cultural groups. One may think about initiating a project to develop different norms for the different multicultural groups for a frequently used test. One may consider initiating this project because of concern that the test is biased against people of color since no, or few, individuals of color were included in the standardization of the test. So, suppose the project develops norms for American Indian clients, norms for white clients, norms for Hispanic clients, norms for Asian clients, and norms for African American clients, and so on. We are sure that the norms for white clients would have the highest scores, while the scores for the other ethnic groups would be lower. Why? Because if the test is developed for one linguistic/social/ethnic cultural group and is administered to members of other cultural groups, without adapting or modifying the test for the other cultures, then the test remains just as biased as when the project began. Thus, having different norms for different ethnic/social/cultural groups presents a professional danger in that in print one could view the various norms as so-called "evidence" that the white clients have the more advanced development. The truth would be lost on many observers; the truth would be that the difference in the norms is not because one group has a level of development superior to other groups, *but because the test is a biased assessment instrument.* Since the test was normed on only one ethnic/cultural/linguistic group, persons with the same characteristics of the standardization group would score the highest on the test. The difference in test scores would not be a reflection of ability, or disability, but rather a reflection of test bias.

**5. Different Cultural Views on Health and Disorder.** The U.S. health care system is characterized by an array of specializations. It is a tendency for persons from the U.S. middle-class to pursue health care to secure professional services for any family member with a disability. The array of specializations typifies the U.S. middle-class view of the person in that in the traditional American cultural view of the body the human body is segmented, or is composed of parts. The body is composed of a number of organ-systems, for example, the digestive system, the respiratory system, the endocrine system, and the social-emotional-affective system. Thus given the loci of the disability, many mainstream families actively and agressively seek out the appropriate specialist for that system, who in turn treats the specific complaint.

Many other cultures possess a more holistic view of the human being, a view that does not segment the body. Therefore, for these cultures the need for, indeed, the existence of, so many specializations can be confusing. If a family member presents with disabilities, making the round of weekly visits with a number of specialists can place tremendous hardship on the family, and, in addition, the family may not be totally in philosophical agreement with the need for various specialists.

It is important to recognize that the way families view disorders, specifically communication disorders, represents a continuum of views about disorders. Some cultures view a disorder as a condition that must be assessed and treated by a certified speech-language pathologist or a certified audiologist. Some cultures view a communication disorder, particularly a speech disorder, as "just the way he talks"; that is, it is noticeable but it is almost regarded as a personality characteristic. Some cultures view disorders as a burden that the family will adjust to and handle. This "continuum" is an extremely simplistic depiction of the range of attitudes about disorder. Families that view disorders as treatable and actively pursue that course of action are the models of service delivery that most disciplines, including audiology and speech-language pathology, are prepared to work with and are confident in their assessment and treatment strategies. Families who do not share this view about disabilities and treatment are often challenges for professionals.

It is also important to recognize that families from ethnolinguistically diverse backgrounds are not monocultural but are bicultural, or actually transcultural. Few families display the values and practices of their traditional cultures. All families share and blend their personal cultural values and practices with traditional cultural values and practices, with the cultural values and practices of their community, and with the cultural values and practices of the larger society.

**6. More Potential For Cultural Conflict In Intervention Setting.** Taylor (in press) submits that clinical practice, such as the fields of audiology and speech-language pathology, is a sociocultural event. Since communication and language are cultural variables, geography, socioeconomic level, and age are examples of sociocultural factors that determine language and communication. Those of us who engage in the diagnosis of communication disorders and the (re)habilitation of communication disorders are engaging in a sociocultural practice. Therefore, when the clinician and the client are from different cultures, the speech-language pathologist must be quite sure that she or he is not diagnosing the presence of communication disorders and engaging in the (re)habilitation of communication disorders based on the clinician's culture, which may not be completely appropriate for the client and family.

**7. Different Service Delivery Preferences.** As discussed above, different cultures have different views regarding health and disorder. One family may expect to and feel comfortable seeking the services of a specialist in communication disorders, that is, an audiologist or a speech-language pathologist. Another family may prefer practitioners from its own culture if the family's views about health and the etiology of disorders differ significantly from mainstream cultural views. Audiology and speech-language pathology service delivery work best when they are community-based and culturally sensitive.

**8. More Linguistic Heterogeneity In Minority Populations.** Individuals who speak more than one language or more than one dialect have a wider range of linguistic behaviors from which to draw; therefore the evaluation of a bicultural and bilinguistic person must be ecologically valid. The term, *ecologically valid assessment,* refers to the need to sample communication behaviors from a number of naturalistic settings and with a number of participants. Conventionally, and traditionally, speech-language diagnostics have taken place in one setting, a clinic, a school speech therapy room, a classroom, an office, or a room in a hospital. Moreover, a basic assumption of diagnostics is that the clinician is sampling representative communication behaviors from the client, because the diagnosis of the communication disorders is based on this sample. Thus a basic assumption of diagnostics is that the communication displayed by the client is representative. For many individuals this may be a secure assumption. However, for ethnolinguistically diverse individuals, this is not a secure assumption. In fact, we feel that more than likely the behaviors that are observed are not representative. Communication behaviors vary with the setting, with the participants, and with the nature of the social event. Multicultural individuals use one communication style when speaking with grandparents, for example, another when speaking with peers, another when interacting with family members, another when communicating with an employer, and another when communicating with a stranger. The diagnostic is the initial contact that the audiologist or the speech-language pathologist has with the client and family, and we are strangers to the family. Children are particularly sensitive to these dynamics of communicative interaction. Ecologically valid assessments are, therefore, of paramount importance because of the linguistic heterogeneity of ethnolinguistically diverse populations.

## CONCLUSION

The fields of audiology and speech-language pathology are exciting professions. The science of diagnosing and treating communication disorders changes constantly, and there is interesting research and clinical procedures constantly evolving. As we enter the next century, the nation's population is changing in terms of age and ethnicity, and the needs of the nation's populations are changing. Audiology and speech-language pathology must respond to the changes and be innovative to meet the challenges that will arise. Our role with ethnolinguistically diverse populations is critical. At the beginning of this chapter we wrote that communication sciences is a field that improves the quality of life for those who receive audiology and speech-language pathology services. Improving the quality of life for individuals from ethnolinguistically diverse populations is very important. Communication is a human behavior that is a universal shared by all cultures. The ability to hear and understand the world around you, to speak, and to understand language is valued by all. During this decade audiology and speech-language pathology will be two professions that address the challenges of providing socioculturally competent services to those with communication disorders.

Our role is an expanding one, for we are members of disciplines that relate to a number of other disciplines, such as education, allied health, medicine, social work, and so forth. All professions are facing the challenges of providing effective clinical and educational services to a multicultural population. Effective interpersonal communication is at the center of effective programming for all disciplines. Audiology and speech-language pathology have important roles regarding expanding other professions' ability to provide services within the context of multiculturalism. Effective interpersonal communication is the goal for practitioners in all disciplines. We have an important role in providing a model for all helping professions.

# 2

# Multicultural Participation in the Professions of Audiology and Speech-Language Pathology

As a result of immigration and other factors related to life and culture, people of color are gradually becoming the majority in the United States. Ramirez (1988) states that there are at least 6 states with a school enrollment of 35% or more students of color, and another 12 states in which students of color make up between 25 and 34% of student enrollment. African Americans, Hispanic Americans, Asian Americans, and American Indians represent more than 50% of the population in one U.S. state, in 24 U.S. cities, and in numerous counties. According to Cole (1987), when all people of color are counted, the percentage of culturally different children enrolled in school programs in cities such as Miami, Philadelphia, and Baltimore is 71, 73, and 80%, respectively. By the year 2000, it is expected that one out of every three students will be black, Asian, or Hispanic (Ramirez, 1988). With the changing demographics that face us for the remainder of this decade, it appears reasonable to assume that the multicultural client in school may become a major focus of the caseload of the speech-language pathologist. In spite of the changing demographics of our society, people of color are still vastly underrepresented as audiologists and speech-language pathologists and as members of the American Speech-Language-Hearing Association (ASHA).

In the 1983–1984 academic year, the total number of students of color enrolled in speech-language pathology and audiology programs nationwide was 2,136 (see Table 2–1). The racial group with the largest number of students was African American with 1,392 students while the racial group with the lowest number of students was American Indian. The total number of students of color (2,136) represented a 14% drop from the 1982–1983 enrollment of 2,622 nationwide. By comparison, there was an overall decline of only 6.6% of all students enrolled in speech-language pathology and audiology programs from 1982–1983 to 1983–1984 (Cole & Massey, 1985). Thus, the percentage of decline in the number of students of color was more than double that of all students in speech-language pathology and audiology.

In the following academic year, 1984–1985, total nationwide enrollment of students of color in speech-language pathology and audiology programs remained relatively constant (see Table 2–2). However, on close examination of the enrollment data, there continued to be cause for concern. Of all the students of color enrolled in speech-language pathology and audiology, there was a 16% increase at the master's level, and a 53% increase at the doctoral level; but there was a 10% decline at the undergraduate level. For all students, there was only a 4% decline at the undergraduate level (Council of Graduate Programs in Communication Sciences and Disorders, 1983–1984).

In analyzing the relative proportions of each ethnic group, compared to all students, in 1984–1985, the proportion of African American students remained relatively constant, and the number of Hispanic students increased by 20%, but Asians and American Indians declined by 47% and 31%, respectively. The percentage of students of color relative to all students remained constant between 1983–1984 and 1984–1985 at 8.5% (Cole, 1987).

In the 1985–1986 academic year, there was a 3% decline in total enrollment in speech-language pathology and audiology, but a 9% increase in the total enrollment of students of color (see Table 2–3).

**Table 2–1.** 1983–1984 Minority Students' Enrollment in Speech-Language Pathology and Audiology Programs

|  | Black | Hispanic | Asian | American Indian | Minority Enrollment | Total Enrollment |
|---|---|---|---|---|---|---|
| Undergraduate | 1,041 | 365 | 95 | 45 | 1,546 | 15,910 |
| Master's | 341 | 113 | 88 | 14 | 556 | 8,473 |
| Doctoral | 10 | 9 | 10 | 5 | 34 | 645 |
| TOTAL | 1,392 | 487 | 193 | 64 | 2,136 | 25,028 |

Source: Council of Graduate Programs in Communication Sciences and Disorders (1984). *1983–1984 National Survey.* Minneapolis, MN.

**Table 2-2.** 1984-1985 Minority Students' Enrollment in Speech-Language Pathology and Audiology Programs

|  | Black | Hispanic | Asian | American Indian | Minority Enrollment | Total Enrollment |
|---|---|---|---|---|---|---|
| Undergraduate | 968 | 389 | 8 | 23 | 1,388 | 15,910 |
| Master's | 374 | 188 | 78 | 19 | 659 | 8,243 |
| Doctoral | 45 | 9 | 16 | 2 | 72 | 647 |
| TOTAL | 1,387 | 586 | 102 | 44 | 2,119 | 24,800 |

*Source:* Council of Graduate Programs in Communication Sciences and Disorders (1985). *1984-1985 National Survey.* Minneapolis, MN.

**Table 2-3.** 1985-1986 Minority Students' Enrollment in Speech-Language Pathology and Audiology Programs

|  | Black | Hispanic | Asian | American Indian | Minority Enrollment | Total Enrollment |
|---|---|---|---|---|---|---|
| Undergraduate | 1,091 | 325 | 130 | 24 | 1,570 | 14,608 |
| Master's | 397 | 150 | 92 | 25 | 664 | 8,744 |
| Doctoral | 43 | 7 | 18 | 3 | 71 | 744 |
| TOTAL | 1,531 | 482 | 240 | 52 | 2,305 | 24,096 |

*Source:* Council of Graduate Programs in Communication Sciences and Disorders (1986). *1985-1986 National Survey.* Minneapolis, MN.

There was an increase in the total enrollment of students of color at the undergraduate level, in contrast to the prior academic year. Also in contrast to the prior academic year was the dramatic increase (58%) in the number of Asian students. In that same period, the number of African American students increased by 9%, American Indian students increased by 15%, but Hispanic students declined by 18%. Overall, enrollment of students of color represented 9.5% of the total student enrollment, which is an increase over prior years.

Data reporting the number of undergraduate students of color enrolled in communication sciences and disorders programs for 1990-1991 (Council of Graduate Programs in Communication Sciences and Disorders, 1991) show that the 1,328 students of color represented 8.7% of all students enrolled in speech-language pathology and audiology programs. There were 756 African American students, 453 Hispanic students, 82 Asian Pacific Islander students, and 37 American Indian/Alaskan Native students (see Table 2-4).

There appear to have been 665 students of color enrolled in master's communication sciences and disorders programs in 1990-1991, which represented 7.8% of all students enrolled. There were 356 African

**Table 2–4.** 1990–1991 Minority Students' Enrollment in Speech-Language Pathology and Audiology Programs

|  | Black | Hispanic | Asian | American Indian | Minority Enrollment | Total Enrollment |
|---|---|---|---|---|---|---|
| Undergraduate | 756 | 453 | 82 | 37 | 1,328 | 15,264 |
| Master's | 356 | 216 | 70 | 23 | 665 | 8,525 |
| Doctoral | 48 | 11 | 14 | 2 | 75 | 688 |
| TOTAL | 1,160 | 680 | 166 | 62 | 2,068 | 24,477 |

Source: Council of Graduate Programs in Communication Sciences and Disorders (1991). *1990–1991 National Survey.* Minneapolis, MN.

American students, 216 Hispanic students, 70 Asian Pacific Islander students, and 23 American Indian/Alaskan Native students. An examination of doctoral student enrollment in 1990–1991 indicates that there were 75 students of color; this number represented 10.9% of all students in doctoral programs. Forty-eight African American students were in doctoral programs, as were 14 Asian Pacific Islander students, 11 Hispanic students, and 2 American Indian/Alaskan Native students.

## FACTORS AFFECTING MINORITY PARTICIPATION

One of the major barriers to effective participation in audiology and speech-language pathology as professions by students of color lies with the dwindling enrollment by students of color across the nation during the 1980s in general. This was particularly so with African Americans. The gains in higher education made by African Americans in the 1970s contrast sharply with the decline in the 1980s. The United States Department of Education revealed that there were 26,000 fewer African American students in college in 1986 than in 1980, the peak year for African American student enrollment in the United States. From 1978 to 1988, the percentage of African American students in the nation's graduate population declined from 6.2% of the total student enrollment to 4.8% (ASHA, 1989). As we look at the effects of these diminishing numbers, we find that they impact markedly on the remaining minority population.

A second barrier affecting participation by people of color in speech, language, and hearing as a profession would be related to the retention of students of color in educational programs. Financial constraint is the primary factor affecting the retention of students of color. Indeed, we are all well aware, or should be, of federal constraints of the 1980s and their effects on education programs. During this decade we were overwhelmed with budget cuts, with the elimination of numerous federally funded programs altogether, cuts in student loan funds, and the institution of new tax laws that affected student financial aid. Add these discouraging events to the increasing costs for higher education, and we can understand why the enrollment of students of color into speech-language and audiology programs was difficult, to say the least.

A third barrier affecting participation of students of color in speech, language, and hearing as professions is related to the accessibility of these programs for undergraduate and graduate study. In spite of integration, 80% of all African Americans who *graduate* from colleges and universities today complete their degrees at predominantly black colleges. This remains so even though it is also true that 60% of all African Americans enrolled in colleges and universities today are enrolled in predominantly black colleges and universities. In this regard, where speech, language and hearing programs are concerned, accessibility is a major problem for African American students in particular. Specifically, there are approximately 107 predominantly black institutions of higher learning in the United States. Of these 107 institutions, only 17 offer programs in speech, language, and hearing. Eight of these 17 offer the master's degree, and four of the eight are accredited by the Educational Standards Board of ASHA. The remaining four are at various stages of the accreditation process as of this writing. Howard University is the only one of these institutions that offers the doctorate degree in speech-language pathology. Howard University has graduated more African Americans with the doctoral degree in speech-language pathology than has any other university in the country. In 1987, there were 11 training programs that were identified as having a bilingual emphasis in speech-language pathology. These programs actively recruit and educate bilingual students to work with bilingual populations with communication disorders. These are master's degree programs (Cole, 1987).

Becoming an audiologist or a speech-language pathologist involves more than simply completing college and going to work. The clinical practice of audiology and speech-language pathology requires certification by ASHA and/or state licensure. To obtain certification or licensure in most states requires (1) a master's degree in audiology or speech-language pathology, (2) completion of a 9-month internship (Clinical Fellowship Year-CFY), and (3) a passing score on the National Examinations in Speech-Language Pathology and Audiology (NESPA), which are administered as specialty examinations of the National Teachers Examination by the Educational Testing Service.

It is the assumption of some professionals that the requirement of the NESPA poses the greatest hurdle for people of color and is, as a result, the reason for a low minority membership in the association. This assumption is based on the pass rate results from the NESPA. According to 1991 data on the NESPA (Educational Testing Service, 1990), test-takers from ethnolinguistically diverse backgrounds scored lower on the National Examination in Speech-Language Pathology than did European American test-takers. On the National Examination in Audiology, test-takers from one ethnolinguistically diverse population, the Asian American, scored similarly to the European American test-takers. The mean score for the Native American test-takers was higher than the mean for the European Americans. The other non-European American cultural groups (i.e., the African American test-takers, the Mexican American test-takers, the Puerto Rican test-takers, and the test-takers identifying with other Hispanic cultures) scored lower than the European Americans.

Research has shown (Payne, Anderson, & Cole, 1988) that the differential pass rates are not related to a lack of knowledge, or status of master's programs, but rather to extra-academic factors such as test anxiety, cognitive style differences, and test-taking skills.

To assume that the differential of the pass rate between culturally and linguistically diverse test-takers and white test-takers on the NESPA is the greatest barrier to minority participation in the ASHA is an assumption obviously based on one's lack of experience with students of color, and nonminority education has had a tendency to make these kinds of assumptions throughout our modern day history of education, regardless of the discipline. In our lifelong association with students of color in this discipline, particularly African American students, we have yet to encounter a single student who maintains that he or she was discouraged from becoming a speech-language pathologist or an audiologist because of anticipated difficulties with the NESPA. Even after discussing pass rate numbers with students, they are still not discouraged to the point of changing their major to another discipline.

Many students of color state that they knew absolutely nothing about audiology and speech-language pathology as professions until they were students in college. For the most part, the majority of these students maintain that they were not aware of speech-language therapy programs in their elementary, middle, and high schools. Most do state, however, that during their development from elementary through high school, they had come into contact with persons who had some kind of speech, language, or hearing disorder. Nevertheless, the major problem still seems to be one of awareness/education. Undergraduate students we teach tell us that when talking with fellow students about their college major, they are frequently asked the question, "What is that field about?"

In one view, a secondary factor that adversely affects minority participation in the ASHA is related to the time commitment that is required to become a communication disorders professional. Specifically, obtaining certification and/or licensure requires 4 years of undergraduate school, 2 years toward the master's degree in most places, and a full-time 9-month CFY. In essence, this is a 7-year commitment that can pose a severe financial burden for students of color, and one which might cause some students to change to another profession as a result. In most cases, however, students are not aware of these requirements until they have already chosen their undergraduate major. And again, in our experience, we have not encountered any students of color at our universities who have decided to change their career option as a result of learning the ASHA requirements for becoming a certified audiologist or speech-language pathologist.

The recruitment and retention of bilingual and minority students for the discipline of human communication sciences and disorders was a priority objective in the Long Range Plan of the ASHA that was established in 1983. In support of this objective, the ASHA Office of Multicultural Affairs has made, and continues to make, a valiant effort to stimulate and increase the number of multicultural and bilingual persons into the professions. The workshops, brochures, marketing aids, and technical assistance for people of color are lauded nationwide, and it has been a major source of hope and positiveness for the ASHA members of color. At the same time, however, the inroads made by the ASHA Office of Minority Concerns (recently changed to the Office of Multicultural Affairs) must be met with positive assistance and action. Many students, including students of color, will need financial assistance in a discipline that is going to require 6 years of education. There is a dearth of nonwhite faculty in communication sciences and disorders, comprising only 5.8% of the full-time academic and clinical faculty in speech-language pathology and audiology programs in 1986 (Cole, 1987). In 1990–1991, one hundred minority full-time college and university faculty comprised 5.2% of the full-time faculty in communication sciences and disorders programs (Council of Graduate Programs in Communication Sciences and Disorders, 1991). Data from 1990–1991 show that there were 52 African American faculty, 22 Asian Pacific Islander faculty, 20 Hispanic faculty, and 6 American Indian/Alaskan Native faculty.

Realistically, the diminishing numbers among students of color are not restricted to the disciplines of audiology and speech-language pathology. Throughout the nation, universities report small numbers of students of color in all disciplines. This is a complex problem that our nation must grapple with in the decade of the 1990s, and we will not begin to see some change in these figures until there is an unqualified commitment from the highest levels of government and education.

# 3

# The ASHA and Cultural Diversity

## MULTICULTURAL ACTION AGENDA 2000

The American Speech-Language-Hearing Association (ASHA) has created a comprehensive multicultural plan to be implemented throughout the 1990s and into the 21st century. This plan, Multicultural Action Agenda 2000 (ASHA, 1991), addresses the issue of an ever increasing culturally diverse society and how this will affect our profession. Through this agenda, the ASHA's goal is to promote affirmative action within our profession to keep up with the demands and needs of society. The ASHA has divided this proposal into six areas of concern: (1) membership; (2) leadership involvement; (3) National Office structure and staffing; (4) policies and programs affecting service, education, and research; (5) government and legislative efforts; and (6) public image.

The first area of concern addressed by the agenda is membership within the ASHA. Currently, the percentage of minority members within the ASHA is approximately 4%, which is far below the representation of these minority groups within the U.S. (approximately 25%). The objective of this agenda is to increase the percentage of ASHA minority members to 10% by the year 2000. Some of the actions intended to accomplish this objective are: develop a comprehensive package of career information to be distributed to minority high schools and minority students; establish mentorship programs for minority high school students to interact with professionals within our field; provide technical support to preprofessional and professional education programs; and increase the size and number of scholarships available to minority students.

The second area of concern addressed by the agenda is leadership involvement. The ASHA policies such as LC 1069 and LC 782 require the consideration of minority groups when selecting members to elected offices and the ASHA committees and boards. Furthermore, LC 4583 requires the consideration of minority groups when selecting faculty for educational programs. Therefore, the objective is to assure maximum participation of minority group members within the ASHA committees, boards, special interest divisions, and activities and programs. The agenda proposes several ways to accomplish this goal. Some of these are: conduct periodic leadership training for minority ASHA members to facilitate the development of leadership potential; establish a talent bank of minority members eligible for educational faculty and committee appointments; and encourage participation in special interest divisions within the ASHA. Two additional policies that demonstrate the ASHA's leadership in minority concerns are LC 782 and LC 4270. LC 782 states that "the committee on Nominations of ASHA give due consideration to school speech-language pathologists and audiologists, women, and federally designated ethnic and minority groups in selecting qualified candidates for elected office." Furthermore, it states that "the committee on Nominations anually prepare a demographic table reporting the distribution of members considered for candidacy." LC 4270 states that "no member holding an elected or paid office in ASHA shall hold membership in private clubs that as a policy exclude persons of racial and religious minorities" (ASHA, 1970, p. 16; ASHA, 1983, p. 173).

The third area of concern is National Office Structure and Staffing. As of January 1990, the representation of minority staff members within the National Office was 18%. Only 3% of this group, however, held managerial level positions. Subsequently, the objective is to increase the proportion of minority groups employed by the ASHA in managerial positions, better approximating their representation within society. One way that the ASHA proposes to achieve this goal is by developing a comprehensive affirmative action plan that would promote filling vacancies within the National Office, with special attention to managerial positions. Also, the ASHA will prepare an annual report, available to all members, containing documentation of minority candidate recruitment efforts for managerial positions. Furthermore, the agenda suggests the establishment of a separate office devoted to multicultural affairs. This will provide the ASHA members with a resource for information pertaining to multicultural issues and will also encourage full participation of minority professionals and students in the ASHA activities.

The fourth area of concern is policies and programs affecting service, education, and research. As cultural diversity increases within the United States, so, too, will the need for communication disorder related services for minority populations. It is therefore vital that the professionals in our field are properly educated and prepared to provide service to these populations. Since most research and norms are based on middle-class white subjects, it is critically important to revise these norms based on a more realistic and diverse culture. Hence, the objective in this area is to establish a commitment to sociodiversity within the ASHA, especially in the areas of education, research, and clinical practice. The actions presented to achieve this goal are: establish an award program to recognize achievements and contributions in the areas of research, education, and clinical services related to multicultural populations; distribute information that will inform members of new research, legislature, and technologies pertinent to multicultural populations; and actively encourage federal agencies and university programs to give multicultural topics high priority in their research agenda.

The fifth area of concern in this agenda is governmental and legislative efforts. Government legislation can have a major impact on minority groups. It is therefore vital that the ASHA continues to support legislative and governmental programs that benefit minority groups in the areas of health, education, and human rights. Consequently, the objective for this area of concern is to promote improved health, educational opportunities, and overall quality of life among minority populations. One way that the ASHA proposes to achieve this goal is to monitor legislation, paying particular attention to areas that will affect multicultural populations. Furthermore, special consideration will be given to legislation and programs that directly impact minority individuals with communication disorders and minority students and professionals involved in communication sciences and disorders. Also, it is necessary to engage in coalitions with other national organizations that have similar goals for minority populations. Finally, the agenda proposes to recognize and support federal legislators and legislative bodies that also possess similar goals and objectives.

The last area of concern addressed by the agenda is public image. Because society is becoming increasingly diverse, so, too, is the population in need of services from our field. It is thus essential that the ASHA portrays an image that reflects its commitment to multicultural populations. To accomplish this task, the information and messages that the ASHA distributes must appeal to the various minority populations within our society. Consequently, the objective is for the ASHA to portray a public image that shows recognition of an increasingly diverse society and a commitment to multicultural populations. Some of the actions presented as means to achieve this objective are: develop a communication disorders education package targeted toward specific minority populations for media and community program usage; recruit spokespersons to lecture on topics of communication disorders targeted towards specific minority groups; and ensure that all materials disseminated from the ASHA properly depict the cultural and ethnic diversity of our society.

In conclusion, Multicultural Action Agenda 2000 was officially adopted by the Executive Board of ASHA in February 1991. The ASHA has since established the Multicultural Issues Board to monitor the implementation of the agenda throughout the 1990s and beyond. This agenda is a critical step towards removing the barriers that hinder full minority participation within the ASHA. Ultimately, it will allow professionals a better understanding of societal needs.

## OFFICE OF MULTICULTURAL AFFAIRS

The Office of Multicultural Affairs (formerly the Office of Minority Concerns) was established by the ASHA in 1969 and lies within the National Office structure. The purpose of the Office of Multicultural Affairs is to provide technical support on issues regarding minority professionals and minorities with communication disorders. This objective involves assisting and informing the Executive Director of the ASHA, the ASHA members, affirmative action employers, academic institutions, other professional organizations, and the general public on these issues. Furthermore, the Office of Multicultural Affairs assesses and analyses "policies and practices to determine barriers to minority participation in association activities, barriers to certification and membership of minority professionals, barriers to minority student recruitment and retention, disparities in service to minorities with communication disorders, and discriminatory assessment and intervention of minorities with handicaps" (ASHA, 1985). Finally, the responsibilities of the Office of Multicultural Affairs also include developing and implementing projects directed toward reversing some of these discriminatory barriers and promoting affirmative action. While the Office of Multicultural Affairs is devoted to these objectives, it is imperative that a commitment to minority concerns be made in all areas of the Association and by all professionals within and related to our field.

Lorraine Cole, former director of the Office of Minority Concerns, states that there are four notable evolutionary stages in the ASHA relative to minorities throughout the history of the profession (ASHA, 1985). Dr. Cole refers to the first period as the pre-enlightenment period, which spanned the first 30 years or so of the Association. During that time, the white middle class was regarded as the single referent for normalcy. All sociocultural aspects of communication were regarded as substandard and such speakers routinely became candidates for therapy or "speech improvement" programs. This attitude underwent a change as a result of lobbying efforts by minority members of the Association. A Black Caucus emerged within the ASHA during the 1960s which urged the Association to make a distinction between linguistic differences and communication disorders. They also raised such issues as the use of racially segregated hotel facilities for conventions and about the ASHA officers and staff holding membership in private clubs that discriminate on the basis of race or religion.

In the second stage, like the early civil rights movement, the focus of the ASHA's early minority program was directed toward blacks—black professionals, black students, and blacks with communication differences and disorders. Then, as women, the elderly, and other minority groups entered the civil rights movement at a national level, the scope of the ASHA's minority program also broadened into the third stage.

Finally, when the National Office was reorganized in 1980, the decision was made to redirect the focus of the minority program to be consistent with its original charge to address racial/ethnic minorities. The issues of the other minority groups were assigned to other units within the National Office.

The Office of Multicultural Affairs has had a significant impact on the establishment of a data base on literature in the field that relates to minorities. In the past, this had not been given adequate research concern. Among such research topics are the following: (1) data on the epidemiology of speech, language, and hearing disorders across minority groups; (2) the disproportionally high incidence of otitis media in American Indians; (3) the known effects of sickle cell anemia on hearing and language development; (4) appropriate instruments for assessing speech, langauge, and hearing in minority and bilingual populations; and (5) the exaggerated facial scarring often found among blacks with cleft lip and palate.

It is the hope of minority members of the ASHA across the nation that the National Office will represent the concerns of all of its members. The Office of Multicultural Affairs, through all of its special education programs, is the organ of the Association that is geared toward helping the ASHA best represent its members in a society that is racially, culturally, linguistically, economically, and geographically diverse.

# 4

# The Black Caucus of the American Speech and Hearing Association: A History

*M. Eugene Wiggins*

The origin of the current association, the National Black Association for Speech, Language and Hearing (NBASLH), goes back to the ASHA convention in 1968 in Denver, Colorado. It was at this convention that a group of African American speech-language pathologists and audiologists confronted the officials of the ASHA and raised significant questions about the involvement of African Americans in the Association. The major concern, of course, was that there were no African Americans who were in any decision-making posts involving the Association. No African Americans were members of the ASHA Legislative Council or on its Executive Board. The individuals who raised these questions felt that African Americans, in general, were "invisible" as far as the ASHA was concerned, and they were supported by the African American membership of the Association. It was at this convention that the ASHA Black Caucus was born.

The founding of the ASHA Black Caucus was spearheaded by a small group of outstanding African American professionals who had never been given an opportunity by the ASHA to demonstrate their skills. Among these professionals were: Ronald Williams, Ernest Moore, Vernon Stroud, Charles Hurst, and Orlando Taylor. The mission of these leaders at this time was to make the concerns of the African American membership known to the ASHA so that, in turn, African Americans would become a visible part of the ASHA's working machine.

Additionally, the Black Caucus addressed the issue of African American people with speech, language, and hearing problems and how these problems might be distinguished from those of other ethnic groups. Specifically, there was a concern that Black English Vernacular dialect was traditionally diagnosed as a "disorder," not a "difference," and the Caucus wanted the ASHA to re-think and re-define "disorder" with a deeper understanding and a sensitivity to the dialect spoken by many African Americans.

The Black Caucus, therefore, urged the ASHA officials to do the following:

1. change its white middle-class character at all levels;
2. bring about equal employment, educational, and clinical opportunities for all African Americans; and
3. encourage appropriate research and curriculum revisions in the area of urban language behavior, most of which is Black language, to the extent that more intelligent clinical and educational services can be made available to Black children (Taylor, Stroud, Hurst, Moore, & Williams, 1969, p. 222).

They also presented a resolution at the annual business meeting of the convention that included five major items that focused on administrative policy, employment, curriculum and certification, social, and the establishment of a new position in the National Office entitled Associate Secretary for African American Affairs. These items are summarized below.

## ADMINISTRATIVE POLICY

The Black Caucus urged that the Executive Board take whatever steps necessary to remove overt and covert racism from within and without the Association. One of the major features of the resolution called for the appointment of a African American member of the ASHA to fill the office of Associate Secretary for School-Clinic Affairs. The Caucus justified its proposal by noting that the ASHA's organizational structure was almost all-white with virtually no African American input at the policy-making level of the Association. The resolution was defeated; instead, a statement denouncing racial discrimination was endorsed, but the resolution offered no specific suggestions on how it could be eliminated. The Caucus then issued the following proposal:

ASHA should issue a public statement denouncing racism, no matter in what form it appears, both within and without the profession, and stating that it is committed to taking whatever steps it can to remove this ugly cancer from all phases of professional and nonprofessional life. Further, the organization should express its recognition of and commitment to the concept of cultural pluralism, including differences in lifestyles, aspirations, interests, and language behavior in the society at-large and of ASHA members in particular.

The resolution also stated that the ASHA should incorporate African Americans at every level of the Association, including the Executive Board, national committees, editorial boards, and all federal and state agencies. Further, the resolution asked that all candidates for elected office in the Association publicly state their positions on sociopolitical matters and answer a set of predetermined questions prior to the election process. Also, the resolution stated that officials of the ASHA should refrain from becoming members in private clubs and organizations that practice racial, ethnic, or nationality discrimination.

## EMPLOYMENT

The resolution stated that the ASHA should require all employers who wish to use the services of the Association to certify that they are equal opportunity employers who do not discriminate against anyone to whom they provide service; that they, the ASHA, will support members who speak out aggressively against racism in the workplace; and that contractors hired by the ASHA be required to present statements periodically regarding the racial and ethnic background, and sex, of their employees based on job categories.

## CURRICULUM AND CERTIFICATION

The resolution stated that the ASHA should require all educational programs to include coursework in sociolinguistics with a focus on African American history, black language, its patterns of development, viable strategies for teaching Standard American English as a second dialect, and assume a leadership role in stimulating basic and applied research in these areas.

## SOCIAL

The resolution stated that the ASHA should not hold professional meetings in cities where racial intermingling and diversity in sexual preference are overtly frowned on.

## EXECUTIVE ASSOCIATE SECRETARY FOR AFRICAN AMERICAN AFFAIRS

The resolution stated that the ASHA should establish in its national office a new position entitled Associate Secretary for African American Affairs to implement new programs and policies pertaining to African American students, professionals, and consumers.

Acknowledging that the Association's business had not been conducted in a manner representative of all its members, the Executive Board and the Legislative Council of the ASHA followed up the proposals submitted by the Black Caucus by presenting three resolutions. The ASHA indicated that the first two resolutions were considered enabling resolutions and were approved by the Legislative Council during the ASHA's convention in Chicago, Illinois, in 1969, one year later. The third resolution was submitted by the Committee on Social and Political Responsibility and approved by the Executive Board in December, 1969 (ASHA, 1970). The three resolutions proposed the following:

1. Association Responsibility for Ameliorating Unfavorable Social Conditions: the Legislative Council charged the Executive Board to assume responsibility for removing unfavorable social conditions that work to the detriment of the Association, and that the Committee on Organizational Structure review the Bylaws and Code of Ethics and recommend to the Executive Board Bylaw modifications which correct any contradictions in the current Bylaws.

2. Representation on ASHA Committees to include school clinicians, females, and blacks with regard to geographic area and work setting, and that the nominations of such individuals to committees by the Committee on Committees be given high priority.

3. Administrative Guidelines for Implementing Social and Political Concerns which called for (a) the hiring of minority members which reflect the ethnic mix in the greater Washington, D.C., community; (b) continued appointment of minorities to committees and boards; (c) including the names of individuals for participation on review boards, site visiting teams, and so forth; (d) recruit minority members into the profession; and (e) encourage local speech and hearing agencies to conduct self-examination surveys regarding the delivery of services to minorities and to the poor.

Interestingly, in that third resolution, which the Vice President for Standards and Ethics transmitted to the American Board of Examiners in Speech Pathology and Audiology (this board no longer exists), the issue of including coursework in sociolinguistics as a requirement for the Certificate of Clinical Competence (CCC) was to be *considered* by the Committee on Clinical Standards (now the Council of Professional

Standards) (ASHA, 1970). That consideration was to last for more than 20 years.

One other critical event took place during the Denver convention. Orlando L. Taylor, then an assistant professor in language pathology at Indiana University, and John Michel, a research associate at the Bureau of Child Research at the University of Kansas at Lawrence, debated on the role of the ASHA in social, political, and moral activities. Taylor argued that by the very nature of our being, our connection with the world society, we must necessarily involve ourselves in the social, political, and moral affairs of this community—indeed, this world. To define ourselves strictly within the narrow confines of speech-language pathologists, audiologists, experimental phoneticians, and so forth, is to deny the nature of our humanness, to diminish our role as critical players on the world stage, a stage beset with problems that are indeed manifested in the social, political, and moral fiber of world society. The ASHA, then, as a professional association, should assume an aggressive leadership role for social, political and moral behavior in areas that reflect free speech and assembly and racism (ASHA, 1969b).

Michel countered that the ASHA must assume responsibility only for issues that pertain to the Association's standards on professional competence. By communicating on matters outside of the Association is to falsely assume that we are experts in areas other than our credentials suggest, qualified to speak out on issues other than speech, language, and hearing. Michel argued further that given the international character of the ASHA, consisting at the time of 150 members who lived in other countries, the Association cannot run the risk of becoming involved in the country's social, political and moral issues where its foreign members may not care to become involved in such issues. Individually, members may pursue this course, he argued, but collectively—as an association—the ASHA can ill-afford the risk of alienating its members by becoming engaged in extraprofessional affairs (ASHA, 1969b).

Another significant issue that was directly related to the social, political, and moral concerns within the profession during the 1970s was officials of the ASHA being members of privately owned clubs that denied admission to nonwhites and women. During the 1970 ASHA annual convention in New York, the Committee on Social and Political Responsibility, led by the late Ronald Williams, then Dean of the College of Ethnic Studies at Western Washington State College, led the fight to have the ASHA officials remove themselves as members of private clubs that discriminate against African Americans and women. The committee recommended to the Legislative Council—which it passed as Resolution 42—that no member holding an elected or paid office in the ASHA shall hold membership in organizations that as a policy exclude persons of racial and religious minorities (PDR Steering Committee, 1971).

At that time, Kenneth O. Johnson, then Executive Secretary of the ASHA, was a member in the Kenwood Country Club in Washington, D.C. In April, 1971, the ASHA Executive Board recommended to the Legislative Council that it rescind that resolution. The suggestion was that implementation of Resolution 42 could subject the Association to legal injunction and financial damages. This was the conclusion of the Association's General Counsel, Mr. Lipman Redman. The Board's recommendation was placed on the Legislative Council's agenda for reconsideration during the November, 1971 convention in Chicago (PDR Steering Committee, 1971).

This touched off a wave of criticism in opposition to rescinding Resolution 42. In a letter addressed to the membership of the ASHA, the members for Professional Democracy and Responsibility (PDR) reacted strongly in a letter addressed to the membership of the ASHA:

> Our reaction was one of dismay and disbelief. It seemed incomprehensible that a position of non-discrimination in today's democratic society could possibly subject us to legal injunct ion and financial damages. Sound legal advice has supported our reaction. We have learned that the racially and religiously restrictive covenants of "social" organizations cannot escape the equal protection of the law concept.

Collective objection to rescinding Resolution 42 came from all corners of the Association, including members of the Committee on Social and Political Responsibility, the ASHA Black Caucus, the Caucus on the Status of Women in ASHA, and the Legislative Councilors from New Jersey and New York. Hilton Davis of Newark, New Jersey, PDR legal counsel, on reviewing the resolution and legal opposition to it, concluded that (1) Resolution 42 is valid and enforceable, (2) there exists no cause for judicial intervention, and (3) there are no principles of law on which a complaining member of the Association could successfully rely (Davis, 1972).

During the course of the next year, several ASHA members, as well as several nonmembers of the Association, began to criticize Resolution 42, the Black Caucus, and the practice of the Caucus to hold meetings that were closed to nonblack speech-language patholoists and audiologists. Collective objection to rescinding Resolution 42 came from all corners of the Association, including members of the Committee on Social and Political Responsibility, the ASHA Black Caucus, the Caucus on the Status of Women in ASHA, and the Legislative Councilors from New Jersey and New York. Hilton Davis of Newark, New Jersey, PDR legal counsel, on reviewing the resolution and legal opposition to it, concluded that (1) Resolution 42 is valid and enforceable, (2) there exists no cause for judicial intervention, and (3) there are no principles of law on which a complaining member of the Association could successfully rely (Davis, 1972).

Carolyn Stewart, chairperson of the Steering Committee of the Black Caucus and a member of the Women's Caucus, voiced the need clearly for just such an alliance on the part of the ASHA members who opposed rescinding Resolution 42 and who appreciated the efforts of the Black Caucus. In her letter to her colleagues warning them of political attempts on the part of some ASHA officials to "turn-back-the-clock," she wrote:

> Since the policies of this organization require the support of Legislative Councilors... if we remain within ASHA we must depend on those councilors sympathetic to our cause on cooperative alliance with other members if we are to eliminate institutional racism in this Association and our profession (Stewart, 1971).

This alliance prevailed.

At the meeting of the Executive Board in December, 1970, presided over by Dr. Frank R. Kleffner, then President of the ASHA, the Board agreed that, in order to implement this resolution [42], every paid and elected official of ASHA should sign a statement to the effect that he or she does not hold membership in a private club which excludes persons of racial and religious minorities. The Board directed Jack Bangs, 1971 ASHA President, to send the statement to members of the National Office staff, members of the Legislative Council, and to all nominees for elected office. It is not clear when, but Kenneth O. Johnson resigned his membership at the Kenwood Country Club.

Resolution 42 was not the only major issue that the Black Caucus confronted during the 1970 annual convention to the ASHA. The Office of the Associate Secretary for Urban and Ethnic Affairs had opened in September 1969. Lovenger H. Bowden, formerly Clinical Director of Speech and Supervisor of the Language Laboratories at Howard University, and a doctoral candidate at the University of Maryland in human development and child study, was appointed to that office as Special Assistant for Urban Affairs (ASHA, 1969a). One of the committees with which she was to work was the Committee on Communication Behaviors and Problems in Urban Populations which was chaired by Orlando Taylor. The committee was another result of the drive of the Black Caucus, and was expected to relate closely with Bowden's office.

Between her appointment in September 1969 and November 1970, when the annual convention was held, Bowden had not been provided any funds to carry out her responsibilities, and, therefore, maintained an office that was severely incapable of appealing to the needs of an urban constituency.

The Black Caucus then had to pursue the course of getting the Office of Urban and Ethnic Affairs funded. The impression among Caucus members was that funds were intentionally being withheld to render the office ineffective. It was perceived as a tactic that could not be allowed. The Caucus felt that such behavior was not only unprofessional, but was insulting as well. Certainly, it was—in the very least—insulting to Lovenger Bowden.

Setting aside 2 hours from its Sunday session in New York, the Legislative Council held an open hearing to receive the concerns of several groups who wanted to make their views known to the Council. Ronald Williams informed the Council of the activities of the Committee on Social and Political Responsibility and on the situation in the Office of Urban and Ethnic Affairs. Before the Council concluded its business in New York, it passed a resolution directing the Executive Board to "approve and to allocate: (a) Association funds for the maintenance of the Office of the Associate Secretary for Urban and Ethnic Affairs, and (2) a specific budget of $48,000 for carrying out the duties of the office for the calendar year 1971" The Council also directed the Executive staff to initiate two staff positions in that office (ASHA, 1971b).

Officials of the Executive Board did not respond positively to this directive. They felt that the Council had extended its duties beyond its powers, and this touched off a heated debate on the separation of the policy making Legislative Council and the managerial role of the Executive Board. The Councilors took office on July 1, 1969, and 1970 marked the first full year that the Legislative Council had functioned under the reorganization of the Association. The Council sent a clear message to the Executive Branch that its legislative powers were not to be compromised by the Executive Branch of the Association. Only one African American was among the members of the Council—Harold Powell of South Carolina, chairperson of the Speech-Language Pathology Program at South Carolina State College.

The Legislative Council felt obliged to get the affairs of the Urban and Ethnic Affairs Office (this was the first name given to the Office of Multicultural Affairs) moving and stood by its resolution. Indeed, not only had the Executive Board not allocated funds, it had not officially recorded into the records of the Association the associate secretary's job description. At its winter meeting in February 1971, the Executive Board, under the ASHA President Jack L. Bangs, authorized the Executive Secretary to establish two positions within the Office of the Associate Secretary for Urban and Ethnic Affairs and to develop programs that focused on the delivery of speech, language and hearing services to neglected populations (ASHA, 1971d).

In July 1971, Johnetta Davis was appointed Assistant Secretary for Program Development in the Office of Ethnic and Urban Affairs; later, in September 1971, Joan P. Cummings (now Joan Payne), was appointed Assistant Secretary for Information Services. Dr. Davis came from the faculty of the District of Columbia Teachers College. Dr. Payne came from Ohio State University, where she was an instructor and clinical supervisor.

Having undergone a dramatically slow beginning, the Office of Urban and Ethnic Affairs was dealt another blow on September 1971 when Lovenger Bowden resigned to accept an appointment as chairperson of the Department of Speech at Howard University (ASHA, 1971a). Her replacement, Dr. Aaron Favors, Jr. of Shaw University in Raleigh, North Carolina, did not arrive at the National Office until January, 1972. Without a leader, Johnetta Davis and Joan Cummings were faced with the responsibility of maintaining that office until he arrived.

Meanwhile, the Executive Board presented to the Legislative Council for consideration at its November, 1971 meeting a resolution calling for the establishment of a Liaison Committee with the Black Caucus. The purpose of this Committee was to receive and study communications (matters of mutual concern) for the Caucus and to make recommendations to the Executive Board regarding those concerns. This process would be handled through the Office of the Vice President for Administration (ASHA, 1971c).

During the 1971 Legislative Council meeting in Chicago, additional rather important events took place: (1) a resolution was passed stating that urban language and urban anthropology be included in the list of course material in the core curriculum suggested for the Certificate of Clinical Competence; (2) the responsibility of developing guidelines to implement Resolution 42 was withdrawn from the Executive Board and the Board charged the Committee on Social and Political Responsibility with the job of creating guidelines to implement Resolution 42 and would then be brought to the Legislative Council for full approval; (3) a Committee on the Status of Racial Minorities was established; (4) the Subcommittee on the Status of Women was elevated to full committee status; and (5) four key members of the Black Caucus were made Fellows of ASHA: Charles G. Hurst, Jr., R. Vernon Stroud, Orlando L. Taylor, and Ronald Williams (ASHA, 1972).

During the Black Caucus meetings at the 1971 ASHA convention in Chicago new members were elected to the Steering Committee, which at that time was headed by Carolyn Stewart, and Donn Bailey became President of the Black Caucus. Announcements were mailed to the Caucus members advising them of the dates and times of Caucus and related meetings. It appeared as though the Caucus wanted to address some issues other than Resolution 42 and the Office of Urban and Ethnic

Affairs. Black Caucus members who were not ASHA certified were encouraged to bring transcripts and clinical clock hours to the convention to get assistance in completing ASHA certification and membership applications.

Additionally, the desire in 1971 was to implement a process in which Black Caucus groups could be organized throughout the country. One group had emerged in Michigan in 1970 as the Michigan Speech and Hearing Association Black Caucus. This group organized prior to the development of any guidelines from the national Black Caucus group. It seems that the Michigan group existed for about 1 year.

The Office of Urban and Ethnic Affairs continued to undergo changes. Aaron Favors, Johnetta Davis, and Joan Cummings resigned from that office on August 31, 1972, less than a year after Favors took office. In their letter of resignation to Executive Secretary Kenneth O. Johnson, the three staff members expressed differences in their perception of their positions and responsibilities to persons in urban and ethnic circumstances and the Association's perception of the same:

> While we understand the position that you and the other members of the Executive Board have taken with regard to the extent to which the Association should become immersed in social, moral and political issues as opposed to professional and scientific concerns, we consider that dichotomy to be false. We believe that, for persons in historically neglected populations, questions and issues of a political, social, and oral nature are inextricably intertwined with the questions of communication for social intercourse and communication as a means of survival . . . we gained insight into the pressing need for establishing new priorities and expanding the delivery of services to persons who are members of neglected minority groups, and who have communication handicaps. This in-depth analysis compels us to move toward an isomorphic relation activities. We feel the need to spend more time and energy in building new models with new priorities, and in conducting activities consonant with those models.

Continuing efforts of the Black Caucus were maintaining the existence of Resolution 42, stressing the need for the resolution to be implemented, and lobbying for the ASHA Office of Ethnic and Urban Affairs. To the Black Caucus it seemed as though the Executive Board was attempting to nullify the mandate laid down by the Legislative Council regarding the resolution. By passing the charge to implement the guidelines for Resolution 42 to the Committee on Political and Social Responsibility, it was posited by many that the Executive Board was engaged in stalling tactics against implementing the resolution. Meanwhile, at its meeting in San Francisco, California, at the annual convention in November, 1972, the Legislative Council defeated the resolution submitted by the Executive Board to rescind Resolution 42 (ASHA, 1973b). The 1971 Legislative Council had voted to table the resolution to rescind Resolution 42. In 1972, the Executive Board again presented a resolution testifying to its continued commitment to the Urban and Ethnic Affairs program from which no activity had taken place since Favors and his two staff members had resigned August 31, 1972.

At the 1972 ASHA convention, the Black Caucus met in a church outside the convention hotel. This may have been the last formal meeting of the Black Caucus.

On August 1, 1973, a year after the Office of Ethnic and Urban Affairs was vacated, Dr. John B. Joyner was appointed Associate Secretary of Urban and Ethnic Affairs. The program was taking on its third associate secretary since the office was opened in 1969; no one had held that office for more than 2 years. Joyner came to the ASHA National Office from Indiana University at Bloomington where he was Director for Human Relations. He had also served previously as associate dean of students and held an assistant professorship at the university (ASHA, 1973a).

The next year, in 1973, in Las Vegas, Nevada, the Executive Board's charge to the Committee on Political and Social Responsibility came up for discussion at the ASHA annual convention. The words at the end of the initial resolution, "because of racial and religious minorities ...," were replaced with "because of his/her race or religion." Annette Zaner of New York, a member of the Committee on Political and Social Responsibility, presented a resolution to the Council calling for the Executive Board to respond immediately to the Council request to implement the resolution. E. Zaslow of Maryland followed Zaner with a resolution which included a model form for each elected or paid ASHA official to complete.

Although the Committee on Political and Social Responsibility, the Committee on the Status of Women, and the Committee on the Status of Racial Minorities continued to function, the charge of the Black Caucus was disappearing. It was becoming apparent that the Black Caucus was not as an effective and viable voice from the African American membership of the ASHA as it had been. There were at least three reasons for the Black Caucus ceasing to exist and to no longer hold formal meetings at the ASHA conventions. In the first place, African American membership in the ASHA was extremely small, and it seemed to be pervaded with an attitude of hopelessness: that there was little ground that they could make in their attempts to make headway within the ASHA. Second, the membership and its leaders were too fragmented geographically, making it extremely difficult to get together frequently for the large number of projects that they deemed necessary in order to get the organization off the ground. A third reason might be attributed to the lessening of social and political activism nationally that followed the large gains made by African Americans after the tumultuous era of the middle to the late 1960s. In addition, rumors had begun to circulate that the officials of the ASHA no longer wanted the Black Caucus to use ASHA as a part of its title (that is, the ASHA Black Caucus). This rumor had no impact on the stability of the Black Caucus. There were a handful of members working desperately to keep the Black Caucus in place.

By 1977, Irma Jeter (now Njeri Nuru) was director of the Office of Urban and Ethnic Affairs of the ASHA. At the national convention in 1977, Jeter was responsible for conducting a workshop on minority education for the national body. By the workshop's end, African Americans were still expressing their dissatisfaction with the ASHA and its relationship with and to people of color (Jeter, 1977). They called for an organization to be formed that would be completely separate from the ASHA. One of the recommendations proposed the following:

> Concerned Blacks in the speech and hearing community should meet to consider and act upon the feasibility of building and sustaining a national association of Black speech-language pathology and audiology professionals. (Jeter, 1977, p. 34)

On January 20, 1978, a small group of African American professionals met in the Howard University Department of Home Economics as the Ad Hoc Development Committee (NBASLH, 1992). Those who attended the meeting were Anita DeFrantz, Norma Edwards, Rosemary Jackson, Ernest Moore, Njeri Nuru, Kay Payne, William Simpkins, Ida Stockman, Orlando Taylor, Eugene Wiggins, and Elizabeth Young. On that date the idea for the National Black Association for Speech, Language and Hearing (NBASLH) was born. In April of the same year, the group was joined by Donn Bailey, Ann Covington, Aaron Favors, Njeri Nuru, Robert Martin Screen, and Dorythea Williams at a meeting at the University of the District of Columbia, and the leg work for the incorporation of NBASLH was underway. Njeri Nuru and Eugene Wiggins wrote the NBASLH By-Laws, and Donn Bailey, Njeri Nuru, and Eugene Wiggins incorporated the organization.

# 5

# Beyond the Black Caucus: The National Black Association for Speech, Language and Hearing, the Native American Caucus of the ASHA, and the Hispanic Caucus of the ASHA

## THE NATIONAL BLACK ASSOCIATION FOR SPEECH, LANGUAGE AND HEARING

The National Black Association for Speech, Language and Hearing (NBASLH) is a scientific association that was established in 1978 to meet the needs and aspirations of African American speech, language, and hearing professionals and students; African Americans with communication disorders; and the African American community. The NBASLH is a nonprofit corporation for charitable, scientific, and educational purposes for African Americans and other racial minorities. In the first volume of the association's publication, *ECHO,* in 1979, it was written that NBASLH is dedicated to achieving national dialogue, awareness, and understanding of the communication behaviors and problems of the black people. The *ECHO* also cited that year that the association is concerned with the development of a unified black perspective of speech, language, and hearing with "a common voice that will speak on issues of common concern" (NBASLH, 1979). The NBASLH logo is a symbol of Zaire which means "reach out with the echo of understanding and speak for all to hear" (Ford, 1983).

As discussed in the previous chapter on the Black Caucus, the NBASLH was founded because, following a decade of struggling to advocate and initiate change within the ASHA, members of the Black Caucus recognized the need for another organization for African Americans in communication sciences and disorders, an organization separate from the ASHA. In 1978 there was an assessment of the speed and extent to which African American members could themselves influence the ASHA, an association which involved itself primarily with issues that reflected views held by the country as a whole. It was strongly felt that as a racial minority within the ASHA, African Americans were placed in the position of constantly having to educate and persuade their European American associates of the needs of African American persons with communication disorders and African American professionals. There was the strongly held view that the chores of constant educating and persuading appeared to produce only few changes in comparison to the amounts of time and effort invested. Hence, a number of African American professional in the field, in keeping with their commitment to serve adequately their people, forcibly argued for the establishment of another organization, which was named the National Black Association of Speech, Language and Hearing (Ford, 1983).

The NBASLH was not formed to be an alternative to the ASHA. Throughout its two decades of existence, the NBASLH has often acted as an external force to stimulate changes within the ASHA that reflect the association's commitment to its membership and their concern about underserved segments of the population.

From the conception of the NBASLH in Washington, D.C., the association has been focused on making the NBASLH a viable association. The first organizational meeting was held at Howard University in 1978. One month later the writing of the constitution and bylaws was begun, and the executive staff and the board of directors were elected. The first NBASLH Board of Directors were Ronald Williams, Chair, Dorythea Williams, Secretary, Ann Covington, Chair-Elect, Sam Geralds, Marie Love Johnson, Njeri Nuru, and Harold Powell. The Executive Staff included Donn Bailey, Executive Director; Robert Screen, Deputy Director; and Eugene Wiggins, Administrative Assistant and Financial Manager (Ford, 1983).

The six primary purposes of the NBASLH are:

1. to promote an increase in the number of black speech, language, and hearing professionals;

2. to promote improvement in the quality of speech, language and hearing services to the black communicatively disabled;
3. to promote the research and development on a body of knowledge, on the identification, diagnosis, and treatment of the black communicatively disabled;
4. to solicit and promote financial support for the training of black students in the fields of speech, language, and hearing;
5. to be an advocate for the black communicatively disabled on local, state, and national levels; and,
6. to dissiminate information to the profession and to the public on communication differences and disorders among blacks.

One significant strength of the NBASLH is its successful programs for professionals and students in the fields of speech, language, and hearing. One program is the NBASLH publication, *ECHO*. The first issue of *ECHO* was published March, 1979. A second program is the NBASLH Research Awards program. Awards are given to African American students to support and encourage master's and doctoral research on the speech, language, and hearing of African Americans. The recipient of the NBASLH Research Award receives a monetary award and presents his or her award-winning scientific paper at the annual NBASLH convention (NBASLH, 1979). A third program is the Association Awards. This category of awards is presented to African American professionals who have made outstanding contributions to understanding communication behavior and problems. Two additional NBASLH programs are public information—which refers to the promotion of information on speech, language, and hearing differences and disorders of African Americans among the professions and the public—and advocacy—the promotion of research services, programs and projects to meet the special needs of the African American speech, language and hearing disabled (Ford, 1983).

There are two additional programs that have been well received by the public. One is the NBASLH annual convention, and the other is the annual NBASLH NESPA Review Course. The first NBASLH convention was held in 1979 in Chicago. Conventions have been held annually since 1979 for the purpose of continuing education and the sharing of scientific and technical knowledge (NBASLH, 1979). In response to the difficulty that many professionals have in achieving a passing score on the National Examination in Speech-Language Pathology, NBASLH conducts an annual preparation course. Individuals from across the United States attend the course, and scholars in the field serve as the faculty for the course.

The NBASLH is truly a national association, with 11 affiliates across the United States. The first NBASLH affiliate was established in Mississippi in 1980. That same year the applications from four other states, Michigan, Wisconsin, Louisiana, and Illinois, were in the process of being approved as affiliates by the NBASLH Board of Directors (Ford, 1983). The affiliates participate in the national programs as well as develop their own programmatic goals to address local and state needs.

## THE NATIVE AMERICAN CAUCUS OF THE ASHA

The Native American Caucus held its first meeting at the annual ASHA convention in 1986. The caucus has continued to meet at the ASHA convention each year since 1986. Members of the Native American Caucus include Native Americans who are in the fields of speech-language pathology and audiology and speech, language, and hearing professionals who provide services to Native Americans. The meetings have been focused on discussing concerns, needs, and difficulties they are experiencing (personal communication, Nunnery, 1993).

One topic that has been discussed is the difficulty many Native Americans experience securing a Clinical Fellowship Year (CFY). Upon graduating with their master's degrees, many Native Americans decide to work at reservations or other remote locations to provide communication assessment and intervention services to Native Americans who are communicatively disabled. The remoteness of their positions makes it extremely difficult to do a CFY because a CFY supervisor would have to travel great distances to meet supervisory requirements.

Another concern is that many white clinicians do not use relevant materials with the Native American children to whom they provide communication services. There is also concern about the inappropriate interactional style many white clinicians use when providing services to Native American children. Very often the concepts of the materials are "foreign to what they are accustomed to" (personal communication, Nunnery, 1993).

A third concern is that many children who have been identified as having a communication disorder are not served well. There are many children who are not receiving needed audiological and speech-language pathology services because of the lack of sufficient numbers of audiologists and speech-language pathologists in the area. There are not enough communication professionals willing to work in remote areas.

A fourth, and very important, concern is that many Native Americans are not recognized as being prominent in the fields of audiology and speech-language pathology. There are few leaders in these disciplines who are Native American. The Native American style of behavior is to not put oneself forward, to not promote oneself. This traditional tendency is a cultural style mismatch when compared to the strategies for building successful careers that many non-Native Americans employ to advance their careers and reputations.

A fifth concern deals with the known, but not extensively researched, diversity across Native American tribes. Nunnery (personal communication, 1993) commented that there well may be diversity in the prevalence of communication disorders among tribes. Research studies have reported that otitis media is quite prevalent among Native Americans. The Native American Caucus has discussed whether high prevalence rates occur among all tribes.

A sixth concern of the Native American Caucus is the dearth of research involving communication behavior and communication disorders among Native Americans. There is not enough. At the Caucus meetings, Native American speech, language, and hearing professionals are encouraged to conduct more research and to do more networking within the caucus.

The Native American Caucus began due to the efforts of the American Indian Professional Training Program at the University of Arizona. Alumni of the program have attended the Native American Caucus meetings and have shared the challenges they have experienced in delivering communication disorders services to Native Americans. One challenge is when a clinician begins working in a Native American community, he or she is not always accepted, even if the clinician is a Native American. There is an "insider-outsider" distinction that slows down the community's acceptance of the professional. Several of the alumni reported that this rapport-establishing effort can take years. One's dress is extremely important. Professionals must dress as the people of the community do so that the tribe will accept them.

A Native American Caucus newsletter has been published by the Native American Training Program at the University of Arizona. One major objective of the newsletter is to stimulate research and networking among the Caucus members.

## THE HISPANIC CAUCUS OF THE ASHA

The first meeting of the Hispanic Caucus was held at the 1992 annual ASHA convention in San Antonio. Several Hispanic members of the

ASHA attended an ASHA professional conference titled Adelante!, which was convened September 1991 to discuss the needs of Hispanic professionals and servicing Hispanic clients who are communicatively disabled. After attending this conference, several Hispanic speech, language, and hearing professionals decided to form the Hispanic Caucus. They received the support of Lorraine Cole, who was Director of the Office of Minority Concerns, and Patrick Carney, who was President of the ASHA (personal communication, Heinsen-Combs, 1993).

The organizers had originally thought that the Hispanic Caucus would be for Hispanic speech-language pathologists and audiologists. An initial meeting of the caucus was planned to be held at the 1992 ASHA convention. Announcements of the meeting appeared in ASHA publications and letters were mailed to bilingual speech-language pathologists and audiologists. The response was overwhelming, particularly from non-Hispanics who work with Hispanic populations. The target group for the Caucus was therefore immediately expanded in response to the tremendous interest expressed by many ASHA members (personal communication, Heinsen-Combs, 1993).

The Hispanic Caucus held its first meeting at the 1992 ASHA convention in San Antonio and presented a poster session. There was international attendance at that first meeting; professionals from Puerto Rico and Mexico attended the Hispanic Caucus. International connections are increasing in that speech, language, and hearing professionals from the speech and hearing association in South America have contacted the Hispanic Caucus of the ASHA and have expressed interest in this newly formed professional organization.

Goals for the Hispanic Caucus were raised at the 1992 ASHA convention and in the first issue of the *Hispanic Caucus for Speech-Language Pathologists and Audiologists,* the newsletter of the Caucus. The general goals of the Caucus are:

1. to better represent Hispanic and non-Hispanic professionals serving the Latino community within the disciplines of speech-language pathology and audiology;
2. to ensure Hispanic representation within all levels of the ASHA;
3. to ensure Hispanic representation in all ASHA-sponsored multicultural activities [Note: One need which was expressed in the Hispanic Caucus newsletter is the need for more minority presenters of ASHA papers (Kayser, 1993). It was observed that the 1992 ASHA convention in San Antonio had a record number of minority emphasis presentations, that is, 105, but that the majority of these presentations were not presented by minority professionals;

4. to share acquired knowledge through research and/or clinical experiences for better service delivery to the Latino community;
5. to encourage clinical research in the various areas of communication disorders, as they pertain to the Hispanic community;
6. to develop guidelines/protocols for improved service delivery to our Hispanic parents/clients;
7. to develop a support network of Hispanic professionals to help all clinicians dealing with the daily challenges of working with the Hispanic population;
8. to decrease the isolation experienced by Hispanic and non-Hispanic clinicians serving the Latino community;
9. to serve as a forum for problem-sharing, problem-solving, and professional growth;
10. to develop clinical and research resources appropriate for the Hispanic population and the clinicians who serve them; and
11. to increase awareness of the needs of Hispanics among the professional and the general public. (Hispanic Caucus for Speech-Language Pathologists and Audiologists, 1993, p. 4)

Two activities of the Hispanic Caucus during its first year of organization have been communicating with the Congressional Hispanic Caucus and joining the National Coalition of Hispanic Health and Human Services Organizations.

# 6

# Legal and Ethical Issues in Communication Disorders Affecting Multicultural Populations

Before 1975, the rights of children with handicaps were not protected in terms of their securing an education. Society and school boards of education, in general, did not appear to have a serious concern that children with handicaps acquire an education. As the public at large became more educated about these children, it began to see that the children, in spite of their handicaps, could perform valuable services to their community. With more education, the public began to perceive that a handicap does not prevent one from making contributions to society.

Much of this education attributed to the growth of special education programs in colleges and universities in the early 1970s. The idea for growth and for making the people with handicaps part of society sprung from President Lyndon B. Johnson's "Great Society Program" after the death of President John F. Kennedy. These events formed a springboard for what was to become important legislation. This legislation had a positive effect on youth who were handicapped, and certainly, on children with communication disorders.

## PL 94-142

PL 94-142, the Education for All Handicapped Children Act (EHA), was implemented in 1975. This act was instrumental in advancing the rights of children with disabilities. Its main purpose is to provide children with handicaps "a free and appropriate education with an emphasis on special education and related services designed to meet their unique needs" (Taylor, 1992). The focus of PL 94-142 is primarily on school-age children with handicaps, ages 3 to 21 years. This act provides more federal money to identify and treat children with disabilities. Because many individuals were not receiving an appropriate education and several were excluded entirely from their peers, this act marked significant progress. Subsequently, children with disabilities are assured equal protection under the law and an appropriate education.

There are many guidelines and requirements that are mandated by the federal government to assure that EHA is properly executed. One requirement of PL 94-142 pertains to eligibility. For the child to be eligible to receive services, that child must have a handicap that impacts them educationally. Children categorized as hearing impaired, language impaired, learning disabled (including brain damage, dyslexia, and developmental aphasia), visually impaired, mentally retarded, emotionally disturbed, orthopedically impaired, autistic, or multihandicapped may qualify for these services. Eligibility is dependent on a team of professionals that provide screenings and assessments of the child in many areas pertaining to education. A committee then discusses and decides the appropriate needs of that child. This committee, which decides both placement and programs, is composed of professionals relevant to that child's education. The committee usually consists of the teacher, special education teacher, parents, administrators, and all appropriate specialists.

Another requirement of PL 94-142 is that services be provided in the least restrictive environment. This is significant because many of the children with disabilities who were previously separated or isolated are now mainstreamed into the classroom with their peers. This requires more of a team effort among the teacher, special education teacher, and other relevant specialists. PL 94-142 also requires a written statement of goals and objectives, called the individualized education plan (IEP). The IEP consists of long-term goals, short-term objectives, present performance levels, statement of specific services, duration of services, objective criteria, evaluation procedures, and professionals involved. It is required that parents are given the opportunity to view the IEP and they are urged to attend IEP meetings pertaining to their child. Parents are also required to be notified of any changes in the IEP. The IEP is reviewed periodically to reassess goals and ensure progress.

## PL 99-457

PL 99-457, or Individuals with Disabilities Education Act (IDEA), is an extension of PL 94-142. This act extends the services required in PL 94-142 from 3 to 21 years of age to birth to 21 years of age. Its main focus is early intervention, including infants and toddlers. The areas of concern are cognitive, physical, communicative, and psychosocial. Children who are at-risk for future educational problems are considered for these services. Some examples of at-risk children are those who are born prematurely, born with physical abnormalities, visually or hearing impaired, very low birth weight, or multiple handicapped.

Like the IEP required in PL 94-142, this act requires an individualized family service plan (IFSP). The IFSP is also a written plan containing goals and objectives for the child. Its contents are very similar to the IEP, and this plan is reviewed periodically to ensure that it is continuing to meet the child's needs. These needs must be met by qualified professionals.

## COMMUNICATION DISORDERS VERSUS COMMUNICATION DIFFERENCES

Dialects occur in almost every language throughout the world. These dialects differ from one another in their lexical, phonological, and syntactical systems. The English language, for example, consists of many linguistic variations, including Black English, standard English, Pennsylvania Dutch, and southern English. These dialects exist as a result of historical and social factors and are valid rule-governed systems for the subcultural groups that use them.

The role of the speech-language pathologist regarding social dialects has been an area of controversy over the years. Some speech-language pathologists have denied clinical services to nonstandard English speakers who have requested services. Others, however, have treated social dialects as though they were communicative disorders (Committee on the Status of Racial Minorities, 1983). This confusion seems to revolve around the question of whether nonstandard English is seen as a difference or a disorder.

The American Speech-Language-Hearing Association stated in 1983 that "no dialectical variety of English is a disorder or a pathological form of speech or language. Each social dialect is adequate as a functional and effective variety of English" (p. 23). Because the role of the speech-language pathologist is to serve the communicatively handicapped, the speech-language pathologist must be able to distinguish between dialectical differences and communicative disorders. To accomplish this task, the speech-language pathologist must have certain competencies. Some of these include knowledge of the particular dialect, knowledge of the phonological and grammatical features of the dialect, and knowledge of nondiscriminatory testing procedures (ASHA, 1983). If a speaker of a social dialect has errors in their language not attributable to their dialect, the speech-language pathologist may treat those errors.

Society has adopted standard English for use in media, government, education, business, and in many other areas. Because of the extensive use of standard English, nonstandard speakers may find it necessary to have access to its use. It is thus the position of ASHA (1983), that the speech-language pathologist is permitted to provide elective clinical services to nonstandard English speakers who do not present a disorder. This should be accomplished by providing competency in standard English without risking the integrity of the individual's social dialect. The speech-language pathologist must have a thorough understanding and appreciation of the community and culture of the nonstandard speaker. In addition, the speech-language pathologist must have knowledge of the linguistic rules of the particular dialect.

It remains the priority of the speech-language pathologist to treat those individuals with communicative disorders. However, as our society becomes increasingly diverse, there is a growing need for the speech-language pathologist to be familiar with social dialects. Awareness of these dialects and their linguistic characteristics will assist the clinician in determining whether there exists a disorder or a difference.

ASHA's position on communication differences versus disorders has perhaps resulted in legislative decisions that have impacted communication disorders and cultural diversity. Among these, two legislative decisions are (1) *Lau v. Nichols*; and (2) the Ann Arbor Decision.

## Lau v. Nichols

There have been a number of significant legal and legislative decisions that have influenced issues on cultural and linguistic diversity in the field of communication disorders. One of the most important legislative decisions was *Lau v. Nichols* in 1974. This case argued on behalf of the Fourteenth Amendment to the United States Constitution which guarantees that all citizens receive equal protection under the law. In the case of *Lau v. Nichols*, the Supreme Court ruled in favor of the plaintiffs from San Francisco's Chinatown. The plaintiffs claimed that the absence of programs designed to meet their specific linguistic needs violated their civil rights. Furthermore, they argued that equality of education goes beyond the provision of the same buildings and books to all students but also includes intangible factors such as language. The Chinese plaintiffs claimed that they were deprived of an adequate and equal education because they could not understand the language (standard English) used in the classroom.

*Lau v. Nichols* established unequivocally that the handling of language differences falls within the range of constitutional guarantees pertaining to equal rights and to Civil Rights legislation. This ruling significantly effected the field of communication disorders and the field of bilingual education. Finally, the ruling of *Lau v. Nichols* was significant because it set a precedent for other legal and legislative actions, such as the passage of the Bilingual Education Act of 1976 and the Ann Arbor Decision.

## Ann Arbor Decision

In the summer of 1979, a potentially precedent-establishing ruling was made by a United States District Court judge. This ruling, now referred to as the Ann Arbor Decision gave legal recognition of social dialects, particularly Black English. The case was *Martin Luther King Junior Elementary School v. Ann Arbor School District*. The court case was a result of concerned parents of black preschool and elementary school children living in Ann Arbor, Michigan. The parents felt that their children's use of 'Black English,' 'Black dialect,' or Black vernacular English' created a barrier to their educational progress in general and to their learning to read in particular" (Bountress, 1987). These parents petitioned the court to require the Ann Arbor School Board to adopt a policy in which teachers are more sensitive to the students' native dialect when teaching standard English to black children.

The issue before the court was whether Ann Arbor School Board was in violation of Section 1703 of Title 20 of the United States Code in which educational agencies are required to remove all language barriers that impede children's equal participation in educational programs (Bountress, 1987). Based on the testimony of many experts in sociolinguistics, the court ruled that the School Board did violate Section 1703(f) of Title 20 of the United States Code. Consequently, the court required that Ann Arbor School Board develop a plan that would aid teachers in identifying Black English dialect and to use this knowledge when teaching children how to read standard English. The Ann Arbor School Board responded with a 1-year educational plan, including 20 hours of inservice education and a series of follow-up seminars. Within this plan, there were 11 objectives, which once met, assist the teachers in identifying and appreciating Black English.

It was believed that this decision was a precedent-establishing ruling that would affect many schools throughout the United States. Unfortunately, this may not have had as dramatic an effect as first predicted. Although the teachers may have become more sensitive to the influence of dialect on learning, it is difficult to determine to what extent this affected teaching style and the overall educational experience. The court's ruling did provide recognition of Black English as a true dialect and demonstrated the ability of the legal system to intervene when children's educational rights are disrupted. These events are extremely significant. However, there continues to be a need for more effective educational programs. Educational facilities, especially universities, need to include courses that educate future and current professionals on cultural and ethnic diversity. Furthermore, programs also need to be implemented that educate professionals about social dialects and help them differentiate these dialects from disorders. Finally, new teaching methods need to be developed that allow standard English to be effectively taught while taking into consideration the student's native dialect.

In summary, it is obvious that the Ann Arbor Decision marked a significant legal decision that legitimized Black English. To further progress in this area of concern, it is necessary to change attitudes and barriers through education.

## LIST OF MAJOR LEGISLATIVE ACTIONS

There have been a number of important court decisions made during the decade of the 1970s that have had a significant impact on the field of communication disorders. Essentially, these court decisions cited the Fourteenth Amendment and Title VI as bases for ruling on behalf of plantiffs, and these rulings have served as a model for similar court cases in the field of communication disorders (Taylor, 1986).

Civil Rights Act of 1964, United States Congress, Title VI

Bilingual Education Act of 1968, United States Congress

Public Law 94-142, The Education of All Handicapped Children Act of 1975

Public Law 95-561, The Bilingual Education Act of 1976

For more than a quarter of a century, the ASHA's Legislative Council has proclaimed numerous association policies addressing minority issues. These policies impact the operations of the Association as well as the practice of the professions. To thoroughly understand the evolution of social awareness within the association and, more importantly, to be fully knowledgeable of ASHA's official stance in specific minority issues, all minority-related resolutions that have been before the Legislative Council from 1961 to 1991 are listed below. These include both passed and defeated resolutions (ASHA, 1993).

_____ 1969:

LC 10-69. BE IT RESOLVED, That the Committee on Committees and the Committee on Nominations give high priority to school clinicians, females, and Blacks in making future committee appointments with due regard to representation by geographic area and work setting, and

BE IT FURTHER RESOLVED, That the Committee on Committees and the Committee on Nominations give an annual accounting of their actions with respect to this resolution.

LC 14-69. BE IT RESOLVED, That ASHA assume responsibility for ameliorating unfavorable social conditions that would be to the detriment of our professional relationships and goals, and

BE IT FURTHER RESOLVED, That the Legislative Council charges the Executive Board to take all steps necessary to insure that all ASHA programs, activities, and responsibilities are conducted in a manner consistent with the spirit and intent of this resolution, and

BE IT FURTHER RESOLVED, That the Committee on Organizational Structure review in detail the By-Laws and Code of Ethics and make recommendations to the Executive Board for By-Law modification which will correct any contradictions between this resolution and current By-Laws.

LC 18-69. BE IT RESOLVED, That the following resolution be referred to the Executive Board for consideration.

WHEREAS, The Black Caucus of the ASHA recognizes that Black Americans have been subjected historically to overt and covert racism in the United States, and

WHEREAS, The same group recognizes that certain administrative policies and practices, clinical services, academic training, and research have not adequately met the needs of the Black members of the Association or of the Black community, and

WHEREAS, The Black Caucus believes that institutional practices can be altered only by aggressive programs which are administered by sufficient personnel,

BE IT RESOLVED, That the Legislative Council endorses appropriate funds for the Associate Secretary for Urban and Ethnic Affairs to appoint necessary consultants to execute her duties as the need arises, and, secondly, appropriate funds from the Office of Urban and Ethnic Affairs to hire two administrative assistants for the following purposes—formulate and enforce policies enacted by the Association concerning elimination of discrimination problems generally and employment problems specifically and coordinate all activities of the Office of Associate Secretary for Urban and Ethnic Affairs and prepare periodic reports to all segments of the Association membership.

LC 22-69. BE IT RESOLVED, That the following named persons be awarded the Fellowship of the American Speech and Hearing Association: Madge Hibler Allen (believed to be the first minority member to be named ASHA Fellow), et al.

_____ 1970:

LC 20-70. BE IT RESOLVED, That the Legislative Council direct the Executive Board to approve and incorporate into the records of the Association, the job description of the office of the Associate Secretary for Urban and Ethnic Affairs as drafted by the ASHA Executive Board and included on page 3 of the 1970 Summary Report of the Executive Secretary.

BE IT FURTHER RESOLVED, That the Legislative Council direct the Executive Board to approve and allocate: (1) Association funds for the maintenance of the of office of the Associate Secretary for Urban and Ethnic Affairs, and (2) a specific budget of $48,000 for carrying the duties of the office for the calendar year 1971, and

BE IT FURTHER RESOLVED, That the Legislative Council direct the Executive Board to acquire two staff positions in the office of the Associate Secretary for Urban and Ethnic Affairs that were referred to the Executive Board by the Legislative Council in Resolution 18, 1969.

LC 38-70. BE IT RESOLVED, That the name of Madge Hibler Allen be added to the slate of nominees for Vice President for Standards and Ethics 1972-1974.

LC 42-70. BE IT RESOLVED, That no member holding an elected or paid office in the American Speech and Hearing Association shall hold membership in private clubs that as a policy exclude persons of racial and religious minorities.

LC 43-70. BE IT RESOLVED, That the following statements be added as Part 4 of Section C of the Code of Ethics of the American Speech and Hearing Association: He must not discriminate on the basis of race, religion, or sex in his professional relationships with his colleagues and clients.

1:
LC 1072. RESOLVED, That the Executive Board is directed to continue its efforts in conformance to the current administrative structure to implement an effective Urban and Ethnic Affairs program.

2:
LC 81-75. RESOLVED, That the Legislative Council reaffirm its policy as reflected in Resolution Number 20, 1970; and further

RESOLVED, That the Legislative Council directs the Executive Board to take all necessary actions to assure the maintenance of this policy; and further

RESOLVED, That these established policies be carefully adhered to in present and future reorganization of the Association and its National Office

_____ 1979:

LC 1-79. RESOLVED, That Article XVI of the Bylaws be changed to read as follows:

Article XVI

Discrimination

The American Speech-Language-Hearing Association recognizes discrimination on the basis of race, national origin, religion, age, sex, or handicapping condition to be inconsistent with its goals, purpose, and policies, and with the professional and ethical responsibilities of its Members, Boards, Committees, and Officers.

Therefore, all programs and activities of the Association and its responsibilities to its Members and to society shall be carried out in such a manner as to be consistent with and in adherence to this policy.

LC 2-79. RESOLVED, That Article XI of the Bylaws be changed to read as follows:

Article XI

Conventions

Conventions of the Association shall be held annually at a time and at a place determined by the Executive Board. Conventions shall be held only in establishments in which meetings can be held without discrimination on the basis of race, national origin, religion, sex, age, or handicapping condition. The responsibility for arranging the Conventions shall be shared by the Scientific and Professional Meetings Board and the Executive Secretary.

In case of emergency, the Legislative Council may, by three-fourth votes, and by mail ballot if necessary, cancel the Annual Convention.

3:

LC 60-80. RESOLVED, That the American Speech-Language-Hearing Association (ASHA) discontinue its affiliation with the International Association of Logopedics and Phoniatrics (IALP) if the Executive Board's Resolution (EB 116-80) is not acted upon by the Bylaws Committee of the IALP and a nondiscriminatory policy with regard to race, national origin, religion, age, sex, handicapping condition, or any other basis that is unjustifiable or irrelevant to the need for and potential benefit from such service in not recommended to be incorporated in the IALP Bylaws by November 1, 1981; and further

RESOLVED, That the Committee on Nominations of the American-Speech-Language-Hearing Association urge the International

Association of Logopedics and Phoniatrics (IALP) to investigate the allegations of discriminatory practice by the South African Speech and Hearing Association.

4:

LC 7-82. RESOLVED, That the Committee on Nominations of the American-Speech-Language-Hearing Association give due consideration to school speech-language pathologists and audiologists, women, and Federally designated ethnic minority groups in selecting qualified candidates for elected office; and further

RESOLVED, That the Committee on Nominations annually prepare a demographic table reporting the distribution of members considered for candidacy in the various priority categories.

LC 16-82. RESOLVED, That the American Speech-Language-Hearing Association adopt the position paper in social dialects.

5:

LC 18-83. RESOLVED, That the Committee on Communication Behavior and Problems in Urban Populations of the American Speech-Language-Hearing Association be changed to the Committee on Cultural Linguistic Differences and Disorders of Communication; and further

RESOLVED, That the Committee charge be changed to read as follows:

To determine the role(s) of the speech-language pathologist and audiologist in the evaluation and treatment of communication differences and disorders in persons of varied cultural and linguistic (which also may include social or economic considerations) circumstances which impinge on their communication competence; to disseminate information about such communication differences and disorders; and, to recommend strategies, methods, etc., to address professionally such communication differences.

LC 45-83. RESOLVED, That full consideration be given to racial and ethnic minorities in planning both the curriculum and faculty of all workshops, conferences and institutes sponsored by the American Speech-Language-Hearing Association.

6:

LC 4-84. RESOLVED, That the American Speech-Language-Hearing Association (ASHA) continue its affiliate membership in the International Association of Logopedics and Phoniatrics (IALP); and further

RESOLVED, That ASHA urge IALP, at its 20th Congress in 1986, to amend further its bylaws to include specific references to nondiscrimination in the provision of clinical services and in the education of future professionals with respect to race, national origin, religion, sex, or handicapping condition; and further

RESOLVED, That ASHA urge IALP to investigate, as carefully and fully as possible, any allegations against affiliate members of discrimination on the basis of race, national origin, religion, sex, or handicapping conditions that precludes the admission of otherwise qualified candidates to educational programs or precludes the provision of needed services to children and adults with communication disorders; and further

RESOLVED, That following the 20th Congress of the IALP, ASHA reevaluate the continuation of its affiliate member status based on a reassessment of IALP's demonstrated commitment to nondiscriminatory practices in the provision of clinical services and in the education of future professionals.

LC 25-84. RESOLVED, That the position paper "Clinical Management of Communicatively Handicapped Minority Language Populations" is adopted by the American Speech-Language-Hearing Association.

7:

LC 7-85. RESOLVED, That the Council on Professional Standards consider adding a provision that the requirements for the Certificate of Clinical Competence include specific content on socially, culturally, economically, and linguistically diverse populations. (Defeated)

LC 20-85. RESOLVED, That the American Speech-Language-Hearing Association (ASHA) will not knowingly invest its reserves in any company or enterprise which is understood to do business in or in any way support the country of South Africa so long as it continues its policy of apartheid; and further

RESOLVED, That the Executive Board be charged to monitor ASHA's investments to ensure no investment of Association funds in any company or enterprise which is doing business with South Africa so long as the policy of apartheid is accepted in that country.

LC 25-85. RESOLVED, That the Committee on Career Information and Development, the Committee on Equality of the Sexes in the Profession, the Committee on State-National Association Relationships, and the Committee on the Status of Racial Minorities be continued as heretofore charged and constituted.

LC 27-85. RESOLVED, That the Committee on Political and Social Responsibility be dissolved. (Defeated)

LC 50-85. RESOLVED, That the American Speech-Language-Hearing Association (ASHA) encourage undergraduate, graduate and continuing education programs to include specific information, course content, and/or clinical practicum which address communicative needs of individuals within socially, culturally, economically, and linguistically diverse populations.

8:

LC 26-86. RESOLVED, That the Committee on Cultural-Linguistic Differences and Disorders of Communication be continued as heretofore charged in LC 18-83; and further

RESOLVED, That the Committee be composed of not fewer than six members, including a chair, to serve for terms of three years.

LC 38-86. RESOLVED, That the charge of the Committee on the Status of Racial Minorities be revised as follows:

To investigate the status of racial/ethnic minorities within the Association and the profession and make specific recommendations to eliminate such vestiges of institutional racism that may exist; to encourage racial/ethnic representation and participation in activities and duties that come within the purview of the Association; to obtain information and develop plans and recommendations regarding policies and practices of education, employment and service delivery systems in communication sciences and disorders which affect or discriminate against individuals of racial/ethnic minorities.

9:

LC 17-88. RESOLVED, That the following definition of bilingual competence necessary to provide clinical services be approved by the American Speech-Language-Hearing Association:

Speech-language pathologists or audiologists who present themselves as bilingual for the purposes of providing clinical services must be able to speak their primary language and to speak (or sign) at least one other language with native or near-native proficiency in lexicon (vocabulary), semantics (meaning), phonology (pronunciation), morphology/syntax grammar), and pragmatics (uses) during clinical management. To provide bilingual assessment and remediation services in the client's language, the bilingual speech-language pathologist or audiologist should possess: (1) ability to describe the process of normal speech and language acquisition for both bilingual and monolingual individuals; and how those processes are manifested in oral (or manually coded) and written language; (2) ability to administer and interpret formal and informal assessment procedures to distinguish between communication differences and communication disorders in oral (or manually coded) and written language; (3) ability to apply intervention strategies for treatment of communicative disorders in the client's language; and (4) ability to recognize cultural factors which affect the delivery of speech-language pathology and audiology services to the client's language community; and further

RESOLVED, That the definition be published in the ASHA journal as soon as possible.

LC 18-88. RESOLVED, That the American Speech-Language-Hearing Association oppose legislation to establish an amendment to the United States Constitution to make English the official language.

LC 22-88. RESOLVED, That the Association Advisory Committee, the Committee on Career Information and Development, the Committee on Equality of the Sexes in the Profession, the Committee on

Long Range Planning, the Committee on the Status of Racial Minorities, and the Joint Committee on State-National Association Relationships be continued as heretofore charged and constituted.

LC 23-88. RESOLVED, That the charge to the Committee on Political and Social Responsibility is: In terms of the general purposes of the Association, and the specific directions defined in the Long Range Plan, identify specific social issues of potential significance to the profession which are not being currently addressed, select those of highest priority, and prepare products which describe the nature of each social issue, its relevance to the profession, and possible implications for research and clinical services; and further

RESOLVED, That the Bylaws of the American Speech-Language-Hearing Association be amended to read:

Article VII
Discrimination

10:

The Association shall not discriminate on the basis of race, national origin, religion, age, sex, sexual orientation, or handicapping condition.

11:

LC 32-91. RESOLVED, That the professional association within each of the U.S. territories (Guam, Puerto Rico, American Samoa, Virgin Islands, and the Commonwealth of Northern Mariana Islands) may apply for recognition by ASHA as a state association and that each territory's application be reviewed in the same manner as would be done for any state association; and further

RESOLVED, That ASHA assume a proactive role in the involvement of multicultural professional associations by contacting these associations to inform them of this resolution.

LC 59-91. RESOLVED, That the Honors of the Association are awarded to Orlando L. Taylor (first minority ASHA member to receive the highest association award).

12:

LC 12-92. RESOLVED, That ASHA establish a leadership award in multicultural professional education to recognize professional education graduate programs in human communication sciences and disorders that demonstrate exemplary efforts to increase program diversity and multicultural literacy; and further

RESOLVED, That the first leadership award in multicultural professional education be given in 1993. (Referred to the Executive Board)

LC 44-92. RESOLVED, That the ASHA Code of Ethics as approved in LC 1-91 be amended as follows:

PRINCIPLE OF ETHICS IV

13: Individuals shall not discriminate in their relationships with colleagues, students, and members of allied professions on the basis of race, sex, age, religion, national origin, sexual orientation, or handicapping condition.

# 7

# Language Development in an Ethnolinguistically Diverse Population: Speakers of Black English Vernacular

A review of the research literature on the language development of children of color reveals that the existing studies can be grouped under three different orientations (Thomas, 1983; Valentine, 1971). The earliest orientation is the *deficit* perspective. Within this perspective nonstandard American English dialects and languages were considered substandard and were regarded as incorrect varieties of standard American English dialect. The ideological premise for this view stemmed from misguided notions of anatomic and physiological differences, misguided notions of genetic superiority/inferiority. This orientation toward people of color living in the United States, particularly African Americans, prevailed from 1619 until the 1960s and 1970s.

However, in the 1960s, speech-language pathology became influenced by the field research on American English dialects being conducted by sociolinguists. One major result of the sociolinguistic research being conducted in the 1960s and 1970s was an understanding that the many varieties of American English spoken in the United States are not the result of genetic differences among peoples, but rather, are the result of environmental differences. That is, the language one speaks is the result of one's country of residence, ethnicity, geographical region, education, socioeconomic level, attitudes about language and communication, and so forth. This orientation is the *difference* perspective. The difference perspective has stressed that no dialect or language is superior or inferior to any other dialect or language and that speakers of nonstandard American English dialects and languages speak valid rule-governed linguistics systems.

The *bicultural* perspective presents the view that many members of nonwhite ethnic groups do not find their culture and the dominant European American culture mutually exclusive, and, thus, are simultaneously committed to both cultures. Biculturalization in the United States is reflected by the preference by many to be identified by both their ethnicity and their American heritage, for example, African American, Chinese American, American Indian, or Hispanic American.

Given this bicultural orientation, the clinician must appreciate the diversity that exists across all families regarding cultural views, beliefs, and practices. There is tremendous cultural and linguistic diversity among families and the extent to which a family adheres, for example, to traditional African American values, behaviors, and beliefs; or to traditional Asian American values, behaviors, and beliefs; or traditional Hispanic American values, behaviors, and beliefs varies with each family. The critical key for audiologists and speech-language pathologists to work effectively with ethnolinguistically different families is to do so with respect and with an appreciation of each family's uniqueness (Anderson & Battle, 1993).

Diversity is the hallmark characteristic of America's ethnolinguistically diverse populations. For example, there is considerable diversity related to ethnicity. To illustrate, African American is the largest non-European ethnic group in the United States. Just as white Americans' ethnic origins are from different countries, primarily in Europe, there is no single geographical, cultural or linguistic origin for African Americans. Below are 23 ethnolinguistically distinct African American groups (Valentine, 1971):

*AfroEnglish*

Northern urban U.S. African Americans
New England U.S. African Americans
Southwest U.S. African Americans
Southern urban U.S. African Americans
Southern rural U.S. African Americans
Appalachia African Americans
Sea Islanders
Guyaneses
West Africans
Southern Africans

East Africans
West Indians

*AfroFrench*

Haitian Creole-speakers
Other French West Indians
French Guianans
Louisiana Creoles
West Africans

*AfroSpanish*

Black Cubans
Aruba-Bonaire-Curaçao (A-B-C) Islander *Papiamento* speakers
Panamanians
Black South Americans
West Indians
Canary Islanders

There are a great many intracultural similarities among these subgroupings of African Americans, as well as there being many differences. Such diversity of ethnicity among African Americans is but one factor that is being used here to present the fact that there is no single cultural group known as the African American family. A similar case can be made for all ethnolinguistically diverse populations.

## LANGUAGE DEVELOPMENT

This chapter focuses on the language development of African American children, one population among the array of ethnolinguistically diverse populations in the United States. Before the studies that are to be discussed are presented to the reader, the authors feel that it is important to provide a discussion of the Black English Vernacular dialect, an American English dialect spoken by many African Americans.

### Black English Vernacular Dialect

In the 1941 text, *The Myth of the Negro Past,* Herskovits presented one myth-like statement about African Americans that was widely held for many centuries:

> The amount of African tradition which the Negro brought to the United States, was very small. In fact, there is every reason to believe ... that the Negro, when he landed in the United States, left behind him almost everything but his dark complexion and his tropical

temperament. It is very difficult to find in the South today anything that can be traced directly back to Africa. (p. 3)

It is, of course, preposterous to presume that the Middle Passage, erased the cultural identities of the millions of Africans who were transported to America. The African slaves came from many regions of West and West Central Africa and were uprooted from societies which for centuries had perpetuated highly developed religions; complex systems of law; pride of history and tradition; a high order of arts and crafts, music and dance; a vast oral literature ranging from proverbs to epics; moral and ethical codes; and complex systems of social organization (Courlander, 1963).

One reason for the denial of African survivals in America was the slave era policy of minimizing the chance of insurrection by disrupting tribal and linguistic ties. This was a futile effort toward hindering communication among the slaves. Futile, because the slaves had not come from villages which were isolated entities and therefore would not be able to communicate with Africans from different tribes. On the contrary, it was common practice for individual African communities to specialize in one product; that is, certain villages would be fisheries, others would be primarily agricultural, others would be involved in metallurgy, some would be textile-oriented, and so forth. It was therefore necessary for traders to travel to different communities to obtain goods not produced in their own villages and to learn different languages for the purpose of trade (Herskovits, 1941).

Throughout West and West Central Africa are a number of different languages, all belonging to two linguistic families. Extending in an irregular area across Africa, from Cape Verde to the Highlands of Abyssinia (Ethiopia), were the Sudanic languages. Belonging to Central and South Africa were the Bantu languages. Hence, the apparent linguistic differences between many of the African tribes were primarily on the vocabulary level, while the syntactic level remained similar. Thus, the primary language learning task required of the Africans as they traveled from village to village was one of acquiring vocabularies. Hence, the linguistic differences did not impose a substantial barrier to communication among Africans because of the familial language relationships.

From the middle of the fifteenth century, when Europeans began to journey to the west coast of Africa for trade, it was immediately apparent to the Europeans that it would be an impossible task to learn the great variety of languages they encountered. Dalby (1971) writes that the principal task of language learning therefore fell to the Africans. As succeeding centuries brought traders, merchants, and seamen from various European countries, including Holland, Portugal, Spain, and England, trade languages, or *lingua francas*, developed so the Europeans could communicate with the Africans. Lingua francas were developed, for the purpose of commerce, from linguistic borrowing among the African and European languages as their speakers came into contact with each other.

Being well experienced in operating divergent sets of vocabulary, the Africans' approach to communicating with the various groups of Europeans was the same as their traditional language learning approach. They grafted the European lexicon onto West African syntactic and phonological structures. English became part of the lingua franca during the sixteenth to seventeenth century.

The African/English language combination evolved from a lingua franca to a *pidgin* when Africans were brought to America. The common plantation policy of mixing slaves of various tribal origins forced the rapid adoption of pidgin Black English by the African slaves. This language system continued to develop. As the first generation of Africans was born in this country, Black English evolved from a pidgin to a *creole* language (Dalby, 1971; Dillard, 1972). Creole is a language form created from the combination of two or more languages that becomes the native language, the "mother-tongue," of a generation of speakers. Stewart (1971) discusses an interesting sociolinguistic phenomenon which also occurred. Later, during the eighteenth century, the separation and distinction on the plantation between house, or domestic, slaves and field slaves occurred, and thereby created social and linguistic "class" differences. Domestic slaves gained access to the plantation home and the plantation family, and in a few cases, the privilege to obtain an education. The slaves belonging to the domestic group were in the circumstance to acquire a more standard variety of English than the creole of the field slaves.

In 1949, a reference, *Africanisms in the Gullah Dialect*, by Lorenzo D. Turner, was published. Turner had spent summers on the sea islands of South Carolina and Georgia examining the Gullah dialect (personal communication, William Clement, 1972). The Gullah dialect is regarded as relic Black English for it has maintained much of early Black English vocabulary, syntax, and prosody. Because of the geographical isolation of the islands from the mainland there was limited sustained contact with the Standard English dialect. In the first half of this century when Turner was conducting his research, he discovered 4,000 West African words, as well as "many survivals in syntax, inflections, sounds and intonations" (Garrett, 1966, p. 240). The Gullah dialect continues to exist today, and when one hears the dialect, one is struck by how different it sounds from "mainstream English." I would describe the prosody of the dialect as sounding rather Carribbean-like. During the past several decades, however, the Gullah dialect has become rather acculturated with the language spoken in the coastal areas of South Carolina and Georgia and is therefore losing its distinctiveness.

Examples of African words that are a part of current American English vocabulary include *tater* for potato, which has been found in several West African languages; *biddy,* used to describe a chick, means a bird in Congolese; *jigger* is derived from *jija* which means a bug in six African languages; *yam* is derived from the African word *nyam*; juke box comes from the Senegalese word *juke* meaning a wild time; *gumbu* is derived from the Angloan word *ki-nyombo*; banana comes through Spanish from Guinea. Examples of additional African words that are interwoven into American English are *okra, zebra, jazz, elephant, ebony, oasis, turnip* (Garrett, 1966).

Additional aspects of language were transported from Africa. The Africans came from societies with strong oral traditions and their storytelling traditions also crossed the Atlantic. Historians have revealed that storytelling involved the traditional use of animals and nature. Stuckey (1968) refers to Hughes and Bontemps' works that point out that the folktales of slaves were actually projections of personal experiences and hopes and defeats, symbolically. For example, the role of the rabbit in slave tales was similar to that of the hare in African folk narratives—that of the trickster who shrewdly outwits and gains a victory over some physically stronger or more powerful adversary. The animal tales told by the slaves with Brer Rabbit as the hero had a meaning far deeper than mere entertainment. Brewer (1968) writes that the rabbit actually symbolized the slave himself. Whenever the rabbit succeeded in proving himself smarter than another animal, the slave rejoiced secretly because the rabbit's victory symbolized his own over his master. From the perspective of the white plantation owner and overseer, the Brer Rabbit tales chronicle the adventures of a sly, mischievous rabbit as he skirmishes day after day with the more powerful but comparatively dull-witted wolf, fox, and bear. From the perspective of the slave quarters, these animal folk tales took on a quite different role. The slaves identified themselves with the rabbit, one of nature's weakest animals, while the plantation-owner was seen as the wolf or fox or bear, three of the strongest and most vicious creatures. Through the language of the tales, the slave depicted the plantation owner's society as violent, rapacious, and hypocritical. In many of the tales, not only does Brer Rabbit triumph over his three enemies, he has a hand in causing a violent fate for each one.

There were also storytelling songs which were interconnected by repetition, an African characteristic. The lyrics conveyed themes from the slaves' daily experiences with much repetition, subtle attacks, and accompanying action or demonstration. Alliteration and the fitting of words to the objects described was a successful literary device of Africa which was continued in slave songs (Fisher, 1953). A humorous example is the ballad about the indestructible "Grey Goose" in a simple unrhymed African leader-chorus design. This seemingly ordinary fowl became a symbol of the ability to "take it," that is, to persevere. The alliterative "Lord, Lord, Lord" of the responding chorus expresses amazement, flattery, and good-humored respect for the tough bird:

> Well, last Monday morning
> Lord, Lord, Lord!
> Well, last Monday morning
> Lord, Lord, Lord!

The repetitive song tells of the bird who was *six* weeks a-falling when he was shot; then he was *six* weeks a-finding; and once in the white house, was *six* weeks a-picking; and then *six* weeks parboiling. When on the table, the repetitions continue: The forks *couldn't stick him* and the knife *couldn't* cut him; thrown in the hog pen, he *broke* the sow's jawbone; then in the sawmill, he *broke* the saw's teeth out. The ballad ends with the grey goose being seen flying across the ocean with a long string of goslings, all going "Quank-quink-quank" (Brown, 1953).

With the great migration of African American families from the rural South to the industrial North during the early decades of this century, Black English Vernacular became not only a southeastern United States dialect, it became woven within the linguistic fabric of the North and Midwest. Black English Vernacular is now a dialect of American English that is spoken by many African Americans in all parts of the country.

It is important to note that there are many more similarities between Black English Vernacular and Standard American English dialects than there are differences. It is also important to note that, even though these are two different dialects, they are neither unintelligible nor uncomprehensible to speakers of other dialects of American English.

Black English Vernacular is a variety of American English spoken by many, but not by all, African Americans. There are a number of phonological and syntactic features that characterize the dialect. All of these linguistic features are optional in their usage; that is, none of the features is obligatory, as is the *-s* marker on third person singular present tense verbs in Standard American English, for example, *she laughs*. No speaker uses all the Black English Vernacular features, and no speaker uses the features within his or her individual linguistic repertoire at every possible opportunity of usage. For example, multiple negation is one of the syntactic features of Black English Vernacular. A speaker of Black English Vernacular who uses the multiple negation feature would not use multiple negation every time he or she produces a negative sentence. Hypothetically, *She didn't want no dessert* as well as *She can't go anywhere* are sentences that could be produced by the same Black English Vernacular speaker. Likewise, nonrealization of the copula, another syntactic feature of Black English Vernacular, occurs in the sentence *She pretty* and is nonoperational in the sentence *The cat is hungry.* Conceivably, these two sentences could be produced by the same speaker, a speaker of the Black English Vernacular dialect.

The label that we are using to refer to this dialect, Black English Vernacular, is just one of several labels that has been coined. Two other labels are Black English and Ebonics. Many feel that none of the labels is adequate or appropriate.

The Black English Vernacular dialect is a dynamic language system. That is, the dialect is influenced by many variables. One factor is geography, just as are all dialects of American English. Speakers of Standard English in Portland, Maine, do not speak the same as do speakers of Standard English in Baton Rouge, Louisiana; and neither do these speakers sound like speakers of Standard English in Eugene, Oregon. Black English Vernacular speakers in Roxbury, Massachusetts, do not speak the same as do Black English Vernacular speakers in Bristol, Tennessee; and neither speak the same as Black English Vernacular speakers in Chicago, Illinois.

The variable that has most significantly influenced Black English Vernacular is time. From the seventeenth century when Black English was pidgin, to now, the last decade of this millennium, the Black English Vernacular dialect has undergone drastic changes in vocabulary, morphology, syntax, and prosody.

*Bidialectalism* is a term referring to speakers' ability to use both Black English Vernacular and Standard American English. The use of both dialects is determined by the social context of the conversation. Black English Vernacular is an appropriate dialect for nonformal exchanges among individuals familiar with the dialect, while Standard American English is appropriate for more formal exchanges, and also for communicating with speakers of other dialects of American English. Bidialectalism is the ability to use more than one dialect and to do so according to the linguistic requirements of the social context. Many African Americans are bidialectal.

## African American Children

Little research has been conducted to examine early language development of African American children. Many of the studies that have examined the language development of African American children have focused on language acquisition by children who are speakers of Black English Vernacular dialect. One of the most complete compilations and critiques of the research of African American children's language development has been presented by Stockman (1986).

## Semantic Development

In the 1970s and 1980s, Stockman, Vaughn-Cooke, and Wolfram (1982) studied the stages of language acquisition of 12 working-class African American children, from Black English Vernacular speaking homes, who ranged in age from 18 months to 4½ years. The researchers studied the children's acquisition of 17 semantic relation categories. Semantic relation categories refer to words and phrases within a speaker's utterances that convey the meanings of the message. To illustrate, the classic sentences (1) *John is eager to please* and (2) *John is easy to please* will be described. While *John* is the subject (*subject* is a grammatical relation term) of both sentences, in terms of semantic relations, *John* is in a different semantic category with each sentence. *John* is the agent, or the doer of the action, in sentence 1; yet, *John* is the recipient of the action in sentence 2. Semantic relations convey meaning.

Stockman et al.'s analyses revealed that the number and types of semantic relation categories increased as the age of the subjects increased. The researchers found that at least 15 (88%) of the 17 categories were coded by every 4½-year-old child compared to 13 (76%) for every 3 year old. Among the 18-month-old children, just seven (41%) of the 17 categories were represented in the language samples.

This study also included an in-depth analysis of the subjects' acquisition of the static-dynamic dimensions of one particular semantic relation category, the *locative*. As its label suggests, locative is a semantic relation that refers to location. Dynamic locative involves utterances that state location and movement, or change of location. Static locative involves utterances that give the location without any mention of movement. Based on their data, the researchers subdivided both the dynamic and the static categories of locative into four subcategories that refer to location in terms of origin, direction, position, and combination reference (Anderson & Battle, 1993; Stockman et al., 1982). To illustrate, within the dynamic category of the locative, Stockman et al. found utterances referring to *origin (They are going from school); direction (They are going away); position (They are going to the shop; Put it on the table);* and *combined reference,* which means that the utterance contained two or more of the subgroups. These researchers also found utterances referring to the static category of the locative and identified *origin (They are from my school); direction (They are away ); position (They are at school);* and *combined reference* within the static locative category.

One research finding was that, of the eight locative subcategories, dynamic direction was the first one acquired. Another major finding was that the acquisition of subcategories within the dynamic and static categories differed. Specifically, within the dynamic category, the order of acquisition was (1) direction, (2) position, (3) combined reference, and (4) origin. Within the static category, the order of acquisition was (1) position, (2) combined reference, (3) direction, and (4) origin. The detailed acquisition data obtained from the Stockman et al. (1982) study provide excellent information that should be used by speech-language pathologists in their assessment of very young working-class African American children's acquisition of language content (Anderson & Battle, 1993).

Stockman and Vaughn-Cooke (1992) have also reported on their in-depth study of the use of the locative in expressions of movement. The researchers tracked the types and frequencies of locative words used by 4 children. This was a longitudinal study that studied the same children for 18 months, from when they were 18 months of age, through to their three year birthdays. Four research questions were addressed in this study: (1) What types of locative words and verbs are commonly used?; (2) Do they express source (for example, *from, off*), path (for example, *over, around*) and goal (for example, *in, on, with*) category?; (3) Are the children's ages and the order of acquisition of locative words related to their membership in a source, path, or goal category?; and (4) Do the inventories of source, path, and goal words and their frequencies of use change as the child develops? From this study Stockman and Vaughn-Cooke found that the types of words the children used to talk about movement changed as they grew older. Source and path words were used most frequently at the earliest ages, while goal words predominated over source and path words at the oldest ages the researchers studied.

One significance of this study is that the researchers found results similar to those reached by other researchers, researchers who studied the semantic development of white, middle-class children. The subjects in this Stockman and Vaughn-Cooke study were African American children from low socioeconomic backgrounds who were acquiring a nonstandard dialect of American English-Black English Vernacular. The researchers wrote that one would not usually expect to find developmental differences among normally developing speakers of the same language. However, decades of prior research have presented African American children as performing below the age or grade levels of white children on various psychometric tests. This study by Stockman and Vaughn-Cooke is different. Their research indicates that African American children who speak Black English Vernacular are acquiring just as rich a linguistic system as are children who are acquiring other dialects of American English.

We encourage students who are interested in studying the morphological, syntactic, and pragmatic linguistic development of African American children to read Stockman's 1986 article that is cited in the References. Stockman has compiled the existing research up to 1986 and presents an analysis of the various studies for the reader. This article is important because Stockman gathered several significant, yet unpublished, studies. Stockman provides several developmental and research implications that stem from her review of the literature. One of her developmental findings is that Black English Vernacular dialectal features begin to appear in the language of young children following the age of 3 years.

For additional discussion of research of the language development of ethnolinguistically diverse populations read the 1993 article by Anderson and Battle. A discussion of the phonological development of African American children can be found in the Iglesias and Anderson (1993) reference cited in the References.

### *Discourse Development*

Heath (1982) has studied the acquisition of conversational competence by children living in three different communities in "Piedmont Carolinas" (Anderson & Battle, 1993). One community described by Heath is a black mill community with rural roots. Within this community children are communicatively competent, and the adults are literate, yet this study reveals discourse development occurring vastly different from how discourse develops within mainstream middle-class family environments.

Current theories of language acquisition stress that language is best acquired in a stimulating environment. In such a context the child's parents provide stimulation that has been described as linguistic input in the context of nonlinguistic support (Bloom & Lahey, 1978). This means that parents' conversation with their young child involves the "here and now," with the object being talked about present and visible, and being manipulated, if possible. The young child who is developing language and the adult display joint attention to the object being talked about. The child is an active participant in this language stimulation event.

Heath's description of the mill community working-class African American's families portrays a different linguistic environment (Anderson & Battle, 1993; Heath, 1982). As infants and preschoolers, these children have no books or toys that are designated as children toys. Viewing this as a deprived and a nonstimulating environment would not take into consideration differing language acquisition approaches in different cultures. The children in this cultural setting acquire language and become communicatively competent. Heath (1982) described that these young children are almost totally in the midst of constant human communication, verbal and nonverbal. Adults in this setting respect and value language and reward children when the children show that they have acquired the ability to use language.

The discourse rules differ from mainstream culture, pragmatics differs, conversational devices differ. Yet these children develop into communicatively competent individuals. One significance of Heath's study is that it helps speech-language pathologists to understand that there is not just one strategy for language acquisition. It also helps us further delineate what aspects of the young child's environment are needed for language acquisition to occur, for example, *warm, caring, and loving human interaction and responsiveness* (Heath, 1982).

Gee (1985) has studied the structure of narratives spoken by children from different sociocultural groups. When studying the structure of narratives, one learns that there are two prevalent styles: topic centering and topic associating. Gee has asserted that working-class children's storytelling styles tend to be a series of utterances that are linked to one another by means of topic associations. Middle-class children tend to produce linear stories centered around a single topic (Taylor, Payne, & Anderson, 1987). These differences in narrative structure can pose difficulty; often the working-class child's narrative is misunderstood. The originality, spontaneity, and structure of the topic associating narrative are often not comprehended and appreciated. Too often the child's story is perceived to be deficient in structure because the structure is different from the topic centering narrative of typical middle-class children's stories. Gee's work is important because he strongly and scholarly rejects the deficit explanation and presents the systematic nature of topic associating narrative structure.

## CONCLUSIONS

We hope that this chapter has provided our readers with an introduction to (1) the Black English Vernacular dialect, and (2) various research studies that have investigated language development among African American children. The studies that are reviewed are only a sampling of the research that exists on the language development of children from ethnolinguistically diverse populations. There still continues to be vast amounts of research needs. Too little is known about language development among other culturally and linguistically diverse populations. For a presentation of the research that has examined the phonological development of Spanish-speaking children, readers are referred to the 1992 article by Iglesias and Anderson that is cited in the References of this text.

Speech-language pathologists are faced with needing to provide competent assessment and intervention services without the confidence of possessing adequate knowledge of language development among many culturally and linguistically diverse populations. Much more research is needed! We hope that this chapter has presented this need in a way that has both provided an understanding of linguistic diversity and has encouraged many students to continue to study culturally and linguistically diverse populations, so that each of you can, within the not too distant future, contribute to the research base of our professions.

It is important to recognize that since there is scattered information on the language development of children from ethnolinguistically diverse populations, it is difficult for speech-language pathologists to competently assess whether children of color are adequately acquiring communication or are presenting with a communication disorder. Without knowledge of normal language acquisition for children from all ethnolinguistic groups, the speech-language pathologists must rely on an armamentarium of strategies. *It is critical for the speech-language pathologist to:*

1. appreciate and have respect for all people and cultural values, beliefs, practices, and behaviors different from her or his own;
2. be knowledgeable about cultural and linguistic diversity;
3. commit to continued education, both from self study and from sponsored programs, to become increasingly knowledgeable about multiculturalism;
4. learn to practice nonbiased assessment, using standardized and nonstandardized instruments and approaches;
5. become an agent for change so that inappropriate diagnoses and inappropriate clinical/educational programming do not occur for any child because of biased assessment procedures.

## Education Implications for Children of Color and the Speech-Language Pathologist

The literature presents many instances of questionable and inappropriate educational programming that has occurred and continues to occur for many children of color. Gollnick and Chinn (1990) refer to earlier studies that investigated the disproportionate placement of children of color in special education. One study cited is Dunn's 1968 research finding that 60 to 80% of students taught in classes for the mentally retarded were children of color from low socioeconomic backgrounds.

A second study, the 1973 study by Mercer, revealed that while Mexican American students constituted 11% of the student population in a particular city in California, they were 45.3% of the students in classes for the mildly mentally retarded. Mercer found that African American students were placed in classes for the mildly mentally retarded at a rate three times greater than their numbers in the city-wide school population.

Chinn and Hughes (Gollnick & Chinn, 1990) analyzed the U.S. Office of Civil Rights Surveys of Elementary and Secondary School from 1978–1984. Their findings were:

> While Hispanics are no longer overrepresented in classes for the mildly mentally retarded in the national data, blacks continue to be. They are also overrepresented in classes for the moderately retarded and the seriously emotionally disturbed. American Indians are overrepresented in classes for the moderately mentally retarded and learning disabled. (Gollnick & Chinn, 1990, p. 151)

All who are concerned with this national trend within special education submit that the reasons for this are sociocultural. There is limited knowledge about assessment with multicultural populations, and there is limited knowledge about communication development and learning styles of children of color.

As students beginning your study of communication sciences and disorders, you are becoming aware of the complex and dynamic nature of language. Cummins (1992), who has written a great deal about second language learning in the educational context by students who speak languages other than English, presents the position that there are two levels of language proficiency: conversational proficiency and cognitive academic language proficiency. Students whose first language (L1) is not English can be observed conversing with peers in appropriate ways in everyday face-to-face situations in both L1 and in English (L2). However, in school these students demonstrate literacy skills that are very much below age-appropriate levels in L2, and in many instances, in both languages.

Cummins has proposed a distinction between basic interpersonal communicative skills (BICS) and cognitive/academic language proficiency (CALP). BICS occurs in everyday communicative contexts, while CALP occurs in decontextualized academic settings and involves the manipulation of language. As a part of his position, Cummins describes a continuum of *cognitive involvement* in communicative activities, from Cognitively Undemanding to Cognitively Demanding. He also describes a continuum of *contextual support* available for expressing or understanding communication, from Context Embedded Communication to Context Reduced Communication (Cummins, 1992).

In context-embedded communication, language is supported by a wide range of meaningful paralinguistic and situational cues. Context-reduced communication relies primarily, and at the extreme end of the continuum, exclusively, on linguistic cues to support meaning, and successful interpretation of the message requires knowledge of the language itself. Context-embedded communication is typical of everyday communication outside of the classroom, wherein many of the linguistic demands of the classroom involve communication activities which are closer to the context-reduced end of the continuum (Cummins, 1992).

Cummins's continuum indices provide for four types of communication activities. Two types of communication activity, (1) cognitive undemanding/context embedded and (2) cognitive undemanding/context reduced, represent communicative tasks and activities in which the linguistic tools have become largely automatized, or mastered, and therefore require little cognitive involvement for appropriate performance. Two other types of activities (3) cognitive demanding/context embedded and (4) cognitive demanding/context reduced represent communication tasks and activities in which the communication tools have not become automatized and thus require active cognitive involvement. Cummins presents the examples that persuading an individual that your point of view is correct is a cognitive demanding/context embedded communication activity, and writing an essay for English class is a cognitive demanding/context reduced communication activity. Children who are in bidialectal or bilingual environments are expected to be able to function effectively along both continua; however, speech-language pathologists, educators, and sociolinguists are not yet sure if they, the professionals, completely understand the extent of the linguistic and the cognitive/academic learning tasks many children of color face. We have discussed Cummins's theory because it presents to those of you studying to become speech-language pathologists that there is so much that is not known about the communication requirements of children from ethnolinguistically diverse populations.

The disproportionate placement of children of color in special education classes and the gaps between the achievement levels of European American children and children from many ethnic and socioeconomic groups have to be addressed. Diagnoses and educational placement come about after the child has had a battery of tests administered by a cadre of professionals from various disciplines. Misdiagnosis and inappropriate educational placement can occur from professionals continuing to assess children of color without regard for the students' cultural and linguistic experiences. Nonbiased assessment can correct these trends; the continuation of biased assessment stems from limited understanding and knowledge.

As you become a practicing speech-language pathologist be determined to become a proactive agent of change and improve the knowledge base of your discipline, so all children may receive all of the benefits of appropriate education and feel that the system cares about them.

What is the role of speech-language pathologists? In 1983 the ASHA advanced its position that guides speech-language pathologists in this area. First, speech-language pathologists cannot treat individuals who speak dialects other than Standard American English and persons who speak English as a second language as though they are persons with communication disorders. Second, speech-language pathologists must have knowledge of the linguistic features of the dialects or languages spoken by the children to whom they provide services. We would add that speech-language pathologists must also acquire knowledge about the traditions, values, practices, and beliefs of the ethnolinguistically diverse populations with whom they work. The speech-language pathologist must collaborate with classroom teachers, English as a Second Language (ESL) teachers, special education professionals, and educational administrators to provide a team approach to multicultural assessment and the delivery of education/clinical programs.

As students in communication sciences and disorders, it is imperative that you strive to gain sociocultural competence, so that as you enter the field you will be prepared to provide socioculturally competent communication assessment and intervention services to the children of this country.

# 8

# Counseling Minorities in Communication Disorders

It is important for students who are beginning their study of communication sciences and disorders to learn that when they become practicing audiologists and speech-language pathologists, their professional responsibilities will include counseling clients with communication disorders and counseling their families.

## THE ROLE OF PERCEPTION

We cannot even begin to think about the counseling process, whether it is with people of color or not, until we have become acutely aware that our "perceptions" will form the basis of the success or failure in communication. The more we perceive—in spite of the fact that our perceptions may be inaccurate—the more we are able to communicate. But, first, we must have perceptions. As Webster (1977) states, perception is considered the cornerstone in the foundation of communication. Indeed, as we approach the year 2000, we are all aware of the alarming predictive statistics which indicate that approximately 65% of our school children will be children from culturally and linguistically diverse groups, mainly African American, Hispanic American, Asian American, and Native American. If this is the case, it will mean that it will be from these populations of school children that we will get the bulk of our communicatively disabled population. If we are to work successfully with these children and their families, we must look again at some of our "perceptions," as they will seriously impact the skills we demonstrate as a communicator and as a counselor.

In an effort to solve its problem of retention of its graduate students of color, the authors were invited to a well-known midwestern university. The objective was to get these students to open up and give us their reasons for the poor retention rate of students of color at the university.

One student, an African American male, told us quite frankly that his problems were due to "perception," and it made it very difficult for him to feel comfortable there. As he elaborated, he went on to say that it all caught him by surprise. These were his classmates in the department, and they were all involved in the same struggles as graduate students. They worked together and studied together. More significantly, and as far as he could tell, they respected and liked each other. He had reached the point that he now felt that the bondage of graduate school was not the only thing that brought them together in friendship. The only significant difference between him and them was that he was African American and they were European American. On many occasions, however, they would even remind him that such a difference between them was not really significant at all. For such a long time he was one of "them," and to think of himself as anything less was ridiculous. Frequently, he said, he would ask himself, Can this really be true?

As his graduate career continued, the young man stated that other problems with "perception" continued to emerge and he began to wonder if liking him, as they claimed, was something real or something superficial. For example, he was told on numerous occasions that he did not "sound" like the majority of African Americans they had known. In other words, he began to realize that one of their perceptions of African Americans was that they all spoke Black English. If they did not, there was something uniquely different and curious about them that deserved getting to know. On other occasions, when they would decide that it was in his apartment that there would be a group study session on a particular weekend, they would frequently say to him, "We know you can really do up that fried chicken."

The young African American concluded: "I do not believe for one moment that these statements were made by my classmates in an attempt to be malicious. Moreover, if I had countered each statement with an accusation of racial prejudice, they would have been shocked, I am sure. Nevertheless, these were their perceptions of me, not their friend, but their black friend, because these are their perceptions of blacks."

In the past few years, the ASHA's Office of Multicultural Affairs, under the leadership of former director Lorraine Cole, has addressed this issue of "sensitivity to minorities" in its January professional education workshops, generally held at Sea Island, Georgia. What has been interesting in these workshops, particularly in their "sensitivity sessions," has been the admission by numerous European Americans that they were not aware that they were using language, both in the teaching and in the clinical environment, that was detrimental to student learning and to client confidence.

## SOME QUESTIONS THE SENSITIVE COUNSELOR SHOULD ASK

Even beginning with the interview of a client of color and his or her family, there are some important questions that clinicians should ask themselves. If the clinician does not have an answer to these questions, then the clinician should begin the process of becoming more socioculturally intelligent if the ultimate good is to be reached. Webster (1977), Luterman (1991), and Schenerle (1992) are excellent sources for looking at the whole counseling process in speech-language pathology and audiology. On the other hand, Sue and Sue (1990) give an in-depth approach to counseling of people of color in particular.

### How do People of Color Feel About the Speech/Language Therapy Process?

In a study of the relevancy of speech and hearing facilities to the African American community, Screen and Taylor (1972) found that in a 2-year period (1967–1969), clinics surveyed in this study had a total of 52,849 clients for speech-language therapy, and only 9.3% of that total were African American clients. Though other culturally and linguistically diverse groups were not studied, it is highly possible that the results would have been similar. The authors of the study posit that before one jumps to the conclusion that lack of education, economics, and transportation are the obvious reasons for such poor participation of African Americans, it must be asked to what extent do African Americans and other people of color feel that the services offered by speech-language pathology agencies are of value.

This study was conducted 25 years ago, and we are certain that results just as interesting would be gathered if the study was replicated today. We hypothesize that many individual clinics would report that the number of African American and Hispanic pediatric clients has increased. Service delivery to other ethnic and cultural groups may be extremely low. Service delivery to adults from ethnolinguistically diverse populations today may show similar results.

## Is My Language Usage Influencing Clients of Color?

Too often, a clinician may not succeed with a client and his or her family because of the language and attitude the clinician uses. It is important for the clinician to be professional, respectful, and sensitive when working with all clients. For example, if the clinician uses slang, or "hip" expressions, such as "What's up?" to greet a client, that clinician will be viewed with suspect by the family. The family would view the clinician as superficial and phony. From that point on, there is almost nothing that this clinician would be able to do to reverse the family's initial impression.

The language that is used in counseling families from ethnolinguistically diverse populations, if not used in the context of the person's culture, can either be a forceful weapon that influences behavior, or it can simply "turn the client off." In this regard, a midwestern European American professor in a sensitivity workshop at the ASHA's Sea Island Professional Education Conference reported that she was not having successful relationships with the African American students in her department. When told, however, that her frequent reference to these students using the terms "you people," "girl," and "boy" were a major reason, the professor was still rather perplexed. "But I use these same expressions in reference to white students, and it does not seem to be a problem," the professor said.

It was at the sensitivity session that the professor learned of the reason for African Americans' objection to these terms and, as a result, she felt more confident about approaching these students again when returning to her university.

## Do I Recognize and Accept the Effects of Culture on Speech and Language Skills?

There are those who would argue that a speech, language, or hearing problem is a speech, language and/or hearing problem, and they are the same for any client. A clinician who espouses to this point of view is one who is saying that culture does not have an influence on a client's speech and language skills. This view acknowledges one perspective only, and as long as it is adhered to, it will cloud the clinicians' attempts to find the real reason for an ethnolinguistically diverse child's problem and, therefore, perform the best service.

In an interview with a Hispanic couple, they told us that they were having difficulty with the speech-language pathologist in their child's school because the speech-language pathologist was trying to convince them that their child's problem certainly was a combination of hearing and auditory processing. "But no," they countered. "Our child *is* hearing you. He is not understanding you because his first language is Spanish, not English, and we only speak Spanish at home." Had the speech-language pathologist recognized the impact of culture on this child's communicative skills, this misunderstanding might not have occurred.

### Do I Have Feelings of Guilt or Paternalism That Interfere With My Objectivity in Counseling Linguistically and Culturally Diverse Clients and Their Families?

In counseling clients and families of color, the clinician should not assume that every problem that the family encounters is a result of racism or prejudice. Families from ethnolinguistically diverse populations are more like European American families than unlike them. Families from all cultures in the United States share *many* characteristics; families are more similar than they are dissimilar.

Accordingly, if the clinician has feelings of guilt because he or she believes that the family is a victim of circumstances, then the clinician can overlook some valuable clues that might make the counseling process successful. More importantly, a feeling of paternalism whereby the clinician plays a protective role is a feeling that does little for fostering the kind of independence, assertiveness, and problem-solving abilities that you want all clients and families to be able to use when they are confronted with situations that require these abilities.

## COUNTERING STEREOTYPES

It is important in our counseling of people of color that audiologists and speech-language pathologists have basic understanding of the characteristics of all the populations with whom they work. At the same time, however, audiologists and speech-language pathologists should work hard to be absolutely certain that their knowledge is more than a series of generalizations that the clinician has formed about cultural groups different from his or her own. If these generalizations are not open to change and challenge, they can indeed become stereotypes, and that is something that must not happen.

*Stereotypes* may be defined as rigid preconceptions we hold about *all* people who are members of a particular groups, whether it be defined along racial, religious, sexual, or other lines (Sue & Sue, 1990). The narrowness of the person who uses stereotypes in his or her thinking is that a perceived characteristic of a particular group is attributed to all persons within that group without regard for differences and variations among individuals.

If a clinician is to be helpful to a person of color who is communicatively disabled and to his or her family, stereotypic thinking must be extinguished. The first way to do that is to learn about your own culture. Second, one must learn as much as possible about culture and cultural and linguistic diversity. Third, it is imperative that the audiologist and the speech-language pathologist provide assistance to other professionals whose skills are needed in the diagnosis and habilitation/rehabilitation process but whose effectiveness will be reduced or negated because the professional engages in stereotypical thinking.

## FAMILY CHARACTERISTICS AND CHILDREARING PRACTICES

What could be more important to audiologists and speech-language pathologists when counseling families of color than knowledge of family characteristics and childrearing practices? The family's cultural beliefs and values form the family relationships and childrearing practices. More importantly, where speech and language are concerned, those family values and practices are important for the audiologist and the speech-language pathologist to know.

The following brief descriptions of some ethnolinguistically diverse groups and their family characteristics and childrearing practices can be helpful to the audiologist and speech-language pathologist in an effort to understand the sociocultural differences that impact on the practice of our professions (Anderson & Battle, 1993). It is important that stereotypes and generalizations are not developed from reading these descriptions. Diversity and variation are human phenomena.

### African Americans

The family life and childrearing practices of African Americans are greatly influenced by history (Greathouse & Miller, 1981). Family values and characteristics reflect both an African heritage as well as adaptive mechanisms developed because of the slavery experience in America. These family values include familial interdependence, mutual aid, compassion, adaptability, flexibility, kinship and group survival, and ethnic pride and loyalty.

Over the past decades, the myriad studies of contemporary African American families have focused mostly on perceived weaknesses of the family structure (Dillard, 1983). Quite often, the conclusion of a weak family structure was conceived by researchers who held the nuclear family structure as the one and only standard. African American families have always shown diversity in structure and relationships. The African American family may consist of only a husband and wife; it may be a nuclear family; or it may consist of one parent and child(ren); or it may include extended family members and the nuclear family; or it may consist of grandparent(s) and child(ren). Such diversity in structure should not be interpreted as weakness. Such flexibility and adaptability in family structure are a part of the African American family heritage that has served important survival and stability purposes. The history of the African American family in the United States has fostered the development of strong kinship ties and diverse, yet strong, family structure as sources of survival, strength, and stability for the family. There often is equalitarianism in spousal relationships in most middle-class African American families in that both parents provide income and share child caring and household responsibilities.

African Americans have a high level of aspiration for their children, and most parents urge and encourage their children to get an education. Dillard (1983) writes that the overwhelming majority of African American college students come from low income families and that many of these parents have little high school education, and most have no college education. African American families value achievement, talent, education, and love for their children.

Regarding childrearing, the newborn is received into a household of warmth, humor, and love and is the center of attention (Greathouse & Miller, 1981). The grandmother is often an important significant other in the life of an African American child and is often quite involved in childrearing if she lives in the same household or in the same city. Grandmothers often assist the family by being a babysitter for the infant providing warmth, affection, and a link to the past. Older siblings and other family relatives also take an active part in child care.

African American fathers, in all socioeconomic levels, take a significant role in child care. They are attentive to their children and strive to have excellent relations with them. Many African American parents believe that too much attention spoils the infant and preschooler and will not adequately prepare the child to cope with the realities and disappointments of life.

Naming is another means of cultural transmission and of giving the infant his or her unique individuality. The names given infants in African American families, as in other cultures, are frequently chosen from among the names of important members of the extended family, or created to give the child individual uniqueness. During the past two to three decades, many African American parents have selected names that reflect the African heritage of the family. Many African Americans are given nicknames as children and retain these nicknames throughout adulthood.

Childrearing practices such as feeding, toilet training, and discipline show cross-cultural differences. During infancy, many African American parents place emphasis on feeding the infant. Many African American mothers initiate toilet training earlier than European American mothers and are rigorous in their training. During the preschool years, the child is greatly influenced by parental attitudes and practices. Obedience and respect for parents are required and expected (Greathouse & Miller, 1981). Spankings are often used by African American parents to discipline the young child. Although middle-class parents are more likely to send a child to his or her room or to temporarily restrict the child's privileges as means of punishment than working parents, spankings are likely to be used by both socioeconomic groups.

Childrearing and socialization in the United States have always presented a double challenge for African American parents. They have had to teach their children the realities of being an African American in the United States, and these teachings begin early in the child's life. On the other hand, most African American parents are aware of the need to raise their young children to be comfortable and confident with their blackness. Most parents expose their children at a young age to black dolls, literature, history, music, and African culture.

African Americans presents a great deal of variability regarding these traditional value orientations, family characteristics, and childrearing practices. It is important for speech-language pathologists and audiologists to not generalize this discussion to all African American families. With the practice of speech-language pathology and audiology becoming increasingly family centered, it is necessary for speech-language pathologists and audiologists to program family and child assessment and intervention services within the cultural context and lifestyle of each family (Anderson & Battle, 1993).

## Chinese Americans

For thousands of years the family has been the basis of Chinese culture and way of living (Char, 1981). Over the course of these millennia, the structure and role of the traditional family has existed without any significant changes. The primary characteristics of the family have been unchanged—patriarchal, patrilineal, extended, located within the broader social organization of the clan and district, and integrated within a system of ethicoreligious beliefs centering around ancestor worship. Characteristics of the traditional Chinese family include the father being the autocratic head of the family and household. The father is responsible for the management of domestic affairs within the household and the behavior of the family members. There has been greater emphasis on the parent-child relationship than on the spousal relationship. A large extended family is another characteristic of the traditional Chinese family. There can be a number of generations living in one home. Chinese social structure has been built on the principle of the extended family (Char, 1981).

Although the Chinese brought their ideal of a large extended family to the United States, they were often unable to achieve the same extended family and clan associations as in China. Therefore, variations of these principles were adopted. Many early Chinese American families lived in Chinese neighborhoods and associated primarily with other Chinese. The people in China exalted the scholar, and in the United States education has always been the means for economic, political, and social advancement. The scholar was considered to be of the highest class and most respected. Chinese American parents expect their children to learn and to do well in school. Early on in the United States it was not unusual for Chinese children to have dual schooling. The children attended Chinese language school after the daily English school. Families insisted on this duality to ensure that the children learned the Chinese heritage, language, and values. Contemporary Chinese American families are often different from earlier Chinese American families. There is frequently a modified extended family wherein the nuclear family resides separately from relatives, while simultaneously maintaining a close relationship between the husband and wife and grandparents.

A quote that describes the Chinese view of childrearing is, "The child is born as a white linen cloth and the design which eventually appears on it is due to the kind of training that he has had" (Char, 1981). Such a tabula rasa philosophy indicates the importance of childrearing in the Chinese culture. The Chinese believe that during the years the child lives with the family, he or she should learn the proper ways of behaving and the values of the family as preparation for his or her future participation in society. The Chinese American family first nurtures and protects the infant, then trains the older child to bring honor to himself and the family. The strategies that the parents employ to teach these values are providing a nurturant environment, definitive statements of sanctioned and nonsanctioned behavior, maximum exposure to models of sanctioned behavior, and restriction from models of nonsanctioned behavior.

Char (1981) reports that the first year of the infant's life is warm and secure. The child is lavished with attention from everyone in the family. A close relationship with the extended family is established if they live nearby. Physical discomfort, such as from a wet diaper or excessive clothing, is immediately corrected. It is not unusual for the infant to frequently sleep in the parents' bed, or in the same room with the parents, or the infant may be allowed to fall asleep in the parents' bed and later carried to his or her own bed. Parents feel that it is more important to provide a strong sense of security at this age and to allay the child's fears than for the young child to show independence.

During the early years the young child is not placed on a rigid toilet training, feeding, or bedtime regimen (Char, 1981). The children eat and sleep according to their own needs, and the mother learns to recognize the child's needs and to take care of them. There often are no structured eating routines. The mother may feed the child mouthfuls of food, such as rice, when she perceives the child as being hungry. In many families, there are no penalties placed on the child for lapses in toilet training until after the child is 4 years of age.

Children are taught behavior and values mainly through observation, participation, and imitation. The parents' sense of complete responsibility plus the belief that the child's behavior reflects his or her training, encourages Chinese parents to keep their children under careful surveillance. The extended family provides models for acceptable behavior. If the parents cannot be accompanied by children, the preference is for one parent to remain home with them. This frequently includes the children accompanying the parents practically everywhere, or the parents limiting their social activities to those to which they can bring children (Char, 1981).

Respect for their parents is a primary virtue taught to Chinese American children. This is manifested by the child's obedience to his or her parents and an attitude of honor and deferense toward them, even when the child is grown and has children. Parents feel totally responsible for their child's behavior, which is considered a reflection on them. If a child misbehaves, he or she has not received proper training at home.

The absence of overt parental praise and reward has been identified as a childrearing practice designed to teach a child humility (Char, 1981). Nonverbal indicators such as a nod of the head or a slight smile are apparent to the child from an early age. Spankings and scolding are common methods of punishment, as well as shaming or lecturing.

Chinese American children are incorporated early and relatively fully into the daily life of the family. They are taught that everyone works for the good of the family. Children are assigned specific tasks and are given a great deal of responsibility at an early age. Older children are responsible for teaching and supervising the younger children and assisting with food preparation. Chinese American family socialization involves the development of strong affective bonds between family members, which helps to make life meaningful during the process of carrying out defined family roles and rules. These bonds are continually emphasized such that an individual's self-esteem and future become significantly bound up with the family and kin (Dillard, 1983).

While there are traditional Chinese American families, there are many families that show varying instances of diversity. Many families incorporate a mixture of traditional Chinese values and European American values as a means of family socialization. It would be incorrect for the speech-language pathologist and audiologist to consider Chinese American families as a homogeneous group (Anderson & Battle, 1993).

## Mexican Americans

There is a strong emphasis on family among the traditional Mexican American family. There is a dedication to the nuclear as well as the extended family, in that there is a close bond between aunts, uncles, grandparents, and cousins (Ehling, 1981). Ehling indicates that first cousins frequently relate to each other as brothers and sisters. The words used to define first cousin in Spanish are "primo hermano" (literally translated, it means *cousin brother*). The aged are highly respected and loved, and children view their grandparents with much affection. Godparents are also important in the traditional Mexican American culture. Much support is gained from this close family relationship; however, such a relationship entails a great deal of responsibility.

The family is likely to be the single most important social unit to Mexican Americans, and personal identification may often be secondary to family identification (Dillard, 1983). Family socialization practices in the traditional sense have a hierarchical structure within the family, that is, increased status and responsibility are extended to older sisters and brothers over younger siblings. The hierarchy also radiates downward from grandparents to parents to children. This traditional Mexican American hierarchy of status within the family contrasts with the equalitarian relationships among family members in European American families.

The role of the father is the one most frequently misrepresented in research literature about the Mexican American family. The Mexican American father is often described as the ultimate authority in all matters. It is true that the husband does have complete authority in most matters; however, he is not a domineering and oppressive force within the family. He does view himself as responsible for the behavior of all family members, and he sees himself as the protector of the family, particularly the women in the family. The wife is expected to be totally dedicated to her family. The mother meets all the nurturing needs of her children and sets the rules by which the children are to live (Ehling, 1981). The birth of a child is a source of celebration. The child is frequently given the name of a saint on whose day he or she was born. The child is given godparents, and a special relationship with the godparents is established.

Many Mexican American families retain use of the Spanish language, and many retain use of traditional medical beliefs and practices. It is believed within the Mexican American culture that to remain healthy one must maintain a balance between hot and cold. It is a traditionally held view that infants are particularly susceptible to the cold and, therefore, are kept tightly bundled. Many health care providers who are inadequately sensitive to cultural differences become distressed by the "overdressing" of the infants when they see the babies dressed in layers of clothing. Another area of dismay for some health care providers who are insensitive to cultural differences is the popular use of the bottle by many Mexican American families. It is not unusual to see a preschooler sucking on a bottle. Mexican American families do not appear to be concerned about early weaning, and for the child, the bottle or pacifier gives a sense of security. Related to feeding, infants are usually fed on demand and picked up when they cry. Children are usually held a great deal, and there is much conversation directed to the infant. Babysitting needs are met by relatives. Table foods are introduced when the baby is about 6 months old and may include bean broth, mashed beans, rice, soups, and eggs.

The young child's world is comprised of cousins, aunts, uncles, grandparents, and other relatives. The young child is treated with much affection by both parents. Discipline for young preschool-age children involves less formal rules being set for them than for many European American children. Non-Mexican Americans may interpret such behaviors as indulging and catering to the children (Ehling, 1981).

There is no single type of Mexican American family; families differ according to their family history, socioeconomic status, politics, geographic location, and degree of assimilation and acculturation. Within this diverse ethnic group, there are traditional and contemporary Mexican, as well as European American patterns of family behavior (Anderson & Battle, 1993; Dillard, 1983).

## Native American

A recent legal definition of the extended Native American family explains that the extended family member shall be defined by the law or custom of the Indian child's tribe or, in absence of such a law or custom, shall be a person who has reached the age of 18 and who is the Indian child's grandparent, aunt or uncle, brother or sister, brother-in-law or sister-in-law, niece or nephew, first or second cousin or stepparent (Farris & Farris, 1981). One feature of the Native American extended family is that all people in the extended family, including the Indian child, are considered equals and have only one horizontal class of relationships. The extended Native American family is an important component in tribal life. Within the Chippewa tribe, the children of one brother are considered the children of another brother. The mother is expected to give birth only every 6 years so that she will be able to properly rear the young child. The father is responsible for teaching the child skills to earn a living, while the child acquires philosophy, religion, knowledge of how to live a good life, and the meaning of things in the world from the grandfather. Frequent repetition of the right way to do things results in producing tribally acceptable social behavior. Storytelling by grandparents often has an educational purpose because the stories have morals that teach what one should do. Neither parent punishes a child. If parents feel that some form of punishment is warranted, an uncle may be given the responsibility of carrying out the task. It is thought that the parents' effectiveness will be reduced should they administer punishment (Dillard, 1983).

The child in the Native American family has traditionally been the one to maintain the customs and traditions of the tribe. Native American belief is that any Native American child is a child of nature and, therefore, a very special person. In the Dakota tribe there is the concept of the Beloved Child. This designation is given to an infant born after a time of great tribal difficulties or tragedy. This child is considered a gift from God and is treated in a special way. The Beloved Child is a symbol of all Native American children because all Native American people have experienced many tragedies and have a special feeling for their children (Dillard, 1983).

The cultural beliefs of the Native American tribe are introduced to the child when he or she is very young. The importance for the individual Native American to be in harmony with nature and to have basic and close spiritual relationships with the environment, for example, water, mountains, trees, earth, is initiated in the early years and is stressed and practiced in Native American child care by the family. To the Native American, the world is regarded as interrelated, and all forms of life are sacred and are to be revered. Children are taught this as a spiritual truth. The child is taught to be as close to nature as possible.

Discipline within Native American families is especially permissive and mild by non-Native American standards. For example, among Pueblo families, there is little need for children to ask "May I?" and there is little need for parents to say "Don't." Parental permission is not a cultural value. Emphasis is placed on developing the child's freedom, responsibility and autonomy (Dillard, 1983). Native American children are well behaved, but are often described by non-Native Americans as overly shy and withdrawn because of the manner in which they conduct themselves in public or away from their families. Farris and Farris (1981) point out that this is not shyness, but the result of conditioning of both adults and children to wait and assess any new situation before they commit themselves and become involved.

Children are also taught that it is inappropriate to discuss one's own accomplishments. Disclosure of one's own strengths may appear as negative behavior among the Native American. Praise is welcome as it is earned, but is usually provided without being sought. Many Native American families do not place emphasis on individualism; cooperative efforts appear to have greater value than individual efforts. Sharing is encouraged not only within a family, but among many families. Possessions as well as duties are shared, and individuals develop a strong sense of belonging. Many families feel that children are competent to care for themselves at an early age and older children are often given the responsibility to supervise younger children (Dillard, 1983; Farris & Farris, 1981).

As stated earlier, the Native American population is a highly heterogeneous cultural group, primarily due to tribal differences. Dillard states that additional factors that account for diversity among Native Americans, in terms of the extent to which they adhere to traditional cultural practices and the extent to which they acculturate cultural patterns of the European American culture, relate to their associations with nature, social systems, various individuals, and world events around them (Anderson & Battle, 1993).

# 9

# Communication Disorders Among Multicultural Populations

It is important to begin this chapter by stating that too little research on this topic has been conducted. Scant and scattered attention has been paid to studying the types and prevalences of communication disorders among populations other than European Americans. Peters-Johnson and Taylor (1986) present important considerations for the examination of communication disorders among multicultural populations. They write, "communication disorders *must* (underlining added) be defined, studied, and discussed from a cultural orientation" (p. 158). Peters-Johnson and Taylor submit that since pathological, or disordered, communication is defined as a deviation from the norm, that norm must be culturally based. To date, the most extensive treatment of this topic to be published is the 1993 text *Communication Disorders in Multicultural Populations* edited by Dolores Battle.

Peters-Johnson and Taylor also cite the 1973 work of Bartel and Grill which submits tendencies for errors of overdiagnosis of the presence of disorders and underdiagnosis of disorders to occur with undesirable frequency with children from non-European American, non-middle-class populations. *Overdiagnosis* refers to the identification of a disorder or problem where none exists; *underdiagnosis* refers to a communication disorder existing but not being identified. One probable basis for errors of overdiagnosis is that the individual is identified as having a speech and/or language disorder from having been administered test(s) that have no persons from multicultural populations, or more specifically, no persons from the individual's cultural and linguistic group among the standardization sample. Another basis for overdiagnosis stems from the standardization sample including persons from multicultural populations, but the standardization sample does not include persons from multicultural populations in adequate numbers or with appropriate representation in all the subgroups of the standardization sample (e.g., all the age groups, all the grade levels).

Peters-Johnson and Taylor submit that underdiagnosis can occur because the assessment procedures employed by the speech-language pathologist are not sensitive enough to detect speech-language disorders because the linguistic standard utilized within the test to detect delayed or disordered communication does not include the client's own linguistic system. Thus, the test cannot validly judge disordered from normal communication development and behaviors for that particular client.

Though the body of literature on communication disorders in multicultural populations is still small, we think it is fair to say that there is improvement in the amount of work that is currently being pursued in this area. The progress in this area is probably due to the prediction that by the year 2000, approximately 65% of the school-age population will be composed of children from diverse cultural backgrounds, that is, African American, Hispanic, Asian, and Native American (Ramirez, 1988). It is predicted that the numbers of individuals from ethnolinguistically diverse populations will continue to increase due to immigration and birth rate patterns so that by the year 2050 more than one third of the nation's population will include ethnically diverse populations.

The authors of this text submit that it is critical for there to be increased exploration of the types and prevalences of communication disorders as presented among multicultural populations because extremely little examination of cross-cultural presentations of communication disorders has occurred. This chapter will first address this topic from a disorder perspective.

## DIFFERING TYPES AND PREVALENCES OF COMMUNICATION DISORDERS

In the late 1960s, when the second author attended her undergraduate alma mater, there were only two communication disorders about which cultural diverse information was discussed. Those two disorders were cleft palate and otosclerosis. This latter communication disorder can result in a hearing disorder. Otosclerosis is a unique bone disease which affects the middle ear and the inner ear (Davis & Silverman,

1978). The most common site of the bony growth is at the oval window wherein the stapes becomes fixed to the oval window. When the stapes is fixed, sound vibrations carried to the stapes from the other two ossicles, the incus and the malleus, cannot be effectively transmitted to the fluid of the inner ear. Otosclerosis is primarily contracted by European American women, and the onset of the disorder is usually during pregnancy.

Regarding cleft palate or orofacial anomaly studies, data contain more cross-cultural information than a number of communication disorders and indicate that pinpointing one factor in the analysis of the cause is virtually impossible. Many factors are speculated as playing a role in the prevalence and incidence of cleft disorders, such as environmental factors (drugs, alcohol, toxic waste, and nutrition), genetic factors, sex, and race. The only way to understand why and how cleft deformities occur is to look at specific cases and analyze the results.

On the basis of several studies conducted, multicultural incidence of cleft lip and/or cleft palate was found to be clearly defined in four races. A review of the literature summarized the results of studies on the four races (Caucasians, African Americans, Asians, and Native Americans). Furthermore, studies conducted in Iran also defined categories of incidence and prevalence of cleft lip and/or palate in their culture with respect to possible influencing factors (Vanderas, 1987).

## Caucasians

When categorizing populations according to race, a significant difference can be found among these various populations. In a 1980 article titled "Blacks With Orofacial Clefts: The State of the Dilemma," Cole provided data that showed that the Caucasian population has a higher incidence of clefts than other ethnic groups, such as African Americans. The Caucasian population showed an incidence of clefts as 1 per 1,099 persons, whereas the African American population showed an incidence of 1 per 1,923 persons. Studies also determined that environmental factors are not as pertinent to the incidence of clefts in the Caucasian population as with other populations. This is particularly true of cultures with lower socioeconomic status (Cole, 1980). In view of this data (.91 to 2.69 cases of clefts per 1,000), it is apparent that the Caucasian population has one of the highest incidence of cleft, with the exception of the Native American population. Since environmental factors such as lower socioeconomic status did not show a significant difference in this group, genetic factors may be a possible area of further study.

Among non-American Caucasian populations, epidemiologic data have revealed a range of 1:1703 in South Africa, according to a 1985 study by Morrison et al., to 1:736 in France, according to a 1982 study by Bonaiti et al., to 1:585 in Sweden, according to a 1972 study by Beckman and Myrberg, (Cole, in press).

## African Americans

The average incidence of cleft lip and/or palate for the African American population appears to range from .18 to 1.67 per 1,000 persons. In two studies (Altemus, 1966; & Myrianthopoulos & Chung, 1974), the ratio of males and females with clefts for African Americans was the same as for the Caucasian subjects; the males outnumbered the females in all cleft types. Although data suggest that the incidence of clefts in African Americans is lower, the physical characteristics of the malformations are more prominent in this population. Defects in nasal structure, deficiency in tissue in the upper lip, and the appearance of postoperative scarring are common to all individuals with clefts, regardless of race. However, the physical makeup of the African American race causes the cleft lip to be more prominent in this population (Cole, 1980). Millard and McNeill (1965) infer that clefts occur more often in lower income groups both in the United States and in Jamaica, where their research was conducted. In their study of African Americans and other mixed ethnic groups, the data claim that the incidence of cleft lip and palate is lower for the Jamaican population. One possible cause for the low incidence in this population in this study may be related to the high infant mortality rate caused by their poor economy.

Further examination of non-American black populations reveal a range of prevalence data for cleft lip and/or cleft palate from 1:8887 in Jamaica, according to the 1965 study by Millard and McNeil, to 1:4404 in South Africa, according to a 1982 study by Kromberg and Jenkins, to 1:2703 in Nigeria, according to the 1981 study by Iregbulem (Cole, in press).

## Asians

Studies of Asians with clefts have concentrated on the Chinese and Japanese populations. Results of the studies on the Chinese population have not been reported with great depth because of the small samples used in these studies. Cole (in press) cites a 1972 study by Emanuel et al. of the prevalence of cleft lip and/or cleft palate among Chinese in Taipei which revealed 1:492, and Fong et al. revealed a 1:500 prevalence in Singapore in 1983.

The Japanese studies reported an incidence of clefts ranging from .85 to 2.68 per 1,000 persons. In 2 studies (Tanaka, 1972; Tsutsui, 1951), the ratio of males and females with clefts showed that males with cleft lip alone outnumbered the females, whereas the other 14 studies showed opposite trends. All of the studies found that males with cleft lip and cleft palate outnumbered females, although females with isolated cleft palate outnumbered males.

## Native Americans

In studies of Native Americans, the range of cleft types among the subjects was .79 to 3.74 per 1,000 persons. The reported incidence of cleft lip with cleft palate was greater than those with isolated cases of either cleft lip or palate. One study (Tretsven, 1963) reported that the ratio of males to females with cleft lip was found to be equal. Furthermore, males outnumbered females in both cleft lip with cleft palate and cleft palate alone.

## Iranians

As a subgroup, Iranians do not typically fall under one of the four categories of diverse cultures that have been specified for this text. Nevertheless, it is a minority culture with respect to the United States. Moreover, the fact that there is research in the literature pertaining to cleft palate in Iran, we think that it is noteworthy to incorporate this information into this section of the text.

A major study on cleft palate incidence was conducted in Iran from 1983–1988 (Abbas, 1992). In the city of Najmeia, clefts exhibited a prevalence of 3.73 per 1,000 live births. The study attempted to isolate hereditary and nonhereditary factors associated with the clefts. The following was revealed: nonhereditary factors associated with clefts were infectious diseases (11.39%), chemical mustard gas (37.97%), dietary deficiency (12.65%), and drug-use during pregnancy (12.65%); hereditary factors associated with clefts revealed a history of malformations in grandparents (18.99%), parents (3.8%), and aunts and uncles (2.53%).

The data from the Iranian study reveal that the incidence of cleft palate in Iran between 1983 and 1988 was higher than any other country in the world. Similar to other studies, the Iranian study showed a higher prevalence of clefts among males than females. Speculation as to why such a high incidence of cleft palate existed in Iran during this period of time usually leads researchers to believe that the high amounts of chemical gas agents used in the Iran/Iraq conflict was a major factor (Abbas, 1992).

# A CROSS-CULTURAL VIEW OF STUTTERING

When looking at stuttering cross-culturally, cultural differences and bilingualism may influence data, thus causing differences in findings from the social majority. By its very nature, stuttering is an extremely diverse area of study in communication disorders. It is a multidimensional problem looking at emotional, behavioral, interpersonal, social, linguistic, cognitive, psychological, and physiologic factors (Shames, 1989). We posit, however, whether communities' perception of stuttering is strongly dependent on culture.

## Attitudes About Stuttering

Attitudes about speech and language disorders tend to vary according to the person's culture. With this in mind, it cannot be assumed that assessment, remediation, and normative data developed for one culture will be appropriate for another. Cheng (1989) states that "professionals need to become cross-culture communicators in order to provide adequate services when working with a culturally and linguistically diverse population" (p. 9).

In looking at attitudes of individuals with communication disorders such as stuttering, studies have shown that North Americans view speech and language disorders as a deficit in communication. Other cultures, however, such as Asians and Native Americans view speech and/or language deficits as indicative of an emotional disturbance in an individual. These varying attitudes can have equally varying effects on the progress and/or improvement of the stutterer, depending on the culture. To be regarded as one who has an emotional "disturbance" could result in abnormal emotional behavior reactions. More importantly, the deficit is often left alone, untreated, and the result is a long-term and serious communication handicap. In another sense, investigation of Japanese and Hispanic cultures regarding stuttering reveals that these two cultures feel that if stutterers "try harder," they would demonstrate much more success in oral communication. As a result, there is little evidence from these two cultures of the importance of speech therapy as a way of improving the stuttering pattern (Bebout & Bradford, 1992).

There are a number of cultural issues that influence stuttering behaviors across different populations. These issues range from such behaviors as: the Japanese male's loss of respect for other males who display fear, to the tendency to deliberately ignore stuttering problems in many African Americans (Shames, 1989).

According to Leith and Mims (1975), there is evidence to support the hypothesis that there does exist a specific behavior difference between African American and European American stutterers. The difference appears to be specifically related to reactions to treatment. African Americans live in a culture where oration is essential. The need to be vocal is evident in the colorful symbolic dialect of African Americans. It is also apparent in the importance placed on entertainment and music, particularly in rap music. For young African American males, a certain rhythmical speech pattern is essential to their existence. The ability to be skilled in this "Black Talk" leads to high prestige and worth. Stuttering behaviors, therefore, for many African American males are sources of ridicule, and they are to be avoided at all cost. In an attempt to maintain his prestige among his peers, the young African American male stutterer may resort to gestures that are also well known to his culture. This behavior makes it difficult to treat the stuttering problem because identification and recognition of the overt behavior can lead to a way of treating the problem. The young African American male is using these behaviors as a way of avoiding the problem, thus making identification and treatment problematic.

In the United States, the prevalence of stuttering ranges from 0.3 to 2.1% in school children from various populations (Van Riper, 1971). Van Riper has written that in many cultures the disorder of stuttering is overlooked because it is not a physical problem. Van Riper (1971) regards this to to be particularly true of the Chinese cultures.

While this discussion of stuttering has focused on cross-cultural variation and has viewed the disorder as capable of being affected by the culture and linguistics of a community, it is important to cite that due to the physiological, as well as the environmental basis of stuttering, this disorder exists among all cultures.

## DOWN SYNDROME IN MULTICULTURAL STUDIES

According to the most recent studies in the literature, there appears to be a higher rate of Down syndrome births in the Hispanic population than in other minority cultures. This increase appears to be related to advanced maternal age for women giving birth in this population. However, when compared to the general population in the United States, there does not appear to be a significant increase in Down syndrome births among Hispanics specifically.

Hook and Harlap (1979) reported that age specific rates of Down syndrome of Asian and North African origins were higher than those of European origin. This study also revealed a higher rate of Down syndrome among Asians and African Americans regardless of maternal age.

Table 9-1 reveals the findings of the study by Hook and Harlap (1979).

The European population used in the study by Hook and Harlap (1979) was derived from the Jewish subculture entirely. At this point, current knowledge about this subculture in regard to communication disorders is almost nonexistent. What does appear to be significant about the findings of Hook and Harlap (1979), however, is that Down syndrome births appear to be related more to maternal age than any other single factor, including culture.

This chapter will now turn to discussing communication disorders among multicultural populations from the viewpoint of age.

## COMMUNICATION DISORDERS AMONG PRESCHOOL POPULATIONS

Due to federal legislation passed in the 1970s and 1980s mandating free and appropriate service delivery for children with disabilities from birth to 21 years of age, there is emerging literature examining cultural diversity. PL 94-142 and PL 99-457 require that children at-risk for developmental disability and children with developmental disabilities be provided services that are socioculturally sensitive and appropriate. With our nation becoming more culturally and linguistically diverse, the greatest evidence of this demographic change is seen among the the country's children. Thirty-six percent of the infants born in the United States in 1984 were born to ethnolinguistically diverse families, and it is estimated that by the year 2000, 38% of the children under 18

**TABLE 9-1.** Rates of Down Syndrome Births in North African, Asian, and European Populations (per 1,000 live births).

| Maternal Ages | North African Down Syndrome Births | Asian Down Syndrome Births | European Down Syndrome Births |
|---|---|---|---|
| 20–24 | 2 | 3 | 1 |
| 25–29 | 7 | 5 | 1 |
| 30–34 | 12 | 9 | 3 |
| 35–39 | 10 | 15 | 4 |
| 40–44 | 11 | 10 | 6 |
| Totals | 42 | 42 | 15 |

*Source:* From Hook, E., & Harlap, S. (1979). Differences in maternal age-specific rates of Down syndrome between Jews of European origin and of North African or Asian origin. *Teratology, 20,* 243–248. Reprinted by permission of Wiley-Liss, A Division of John Wiley and Sons, Inc., copyright © 1979.

years of age will be from non-European American families. Interestingly, as the overall percentage of children in the United States is decreasing, the proportion of children from culturally and linguistically diverse groups is increasing (Hanson, Lynch, & Wayman; 1990). Using a very conservative estimate, Hanson, Lynch, and Wayman estimate that 3% of infants and toddlers from ethnolinguistically diverse populations will be disabled. These authors also estimate that a much larger percentage will be at-risk for disabilities.

At birth many African American infants present with low, and very low, birth weight (Schoendorf, Hogue, Kleinman, & Rowley, 1992). Statistics suggest that African American mothers are two to three times as likely to give birth to infants with low birth weight than are European American mothers. Research studies that have controlled variables such as education, age, and socioeconomic status have persisted in finding that African American babies are born with lower birthweights than European American babies. The significance of these findings is that prematurity is an extremely important factor related to infant developmental disabilities and at-risk status, and low birth weight is a leading cause or characteristic of prematurity. Low birth weight infants are at risk for developmental disabilities which impact on the normal development of communication, disabilities such as brain damage, cerebral palsy, and mental retardation (Anderson & McNeilly, 1992).

African American children account for more than 50% of all children with AIDS. The occurrence of developmental disabilities in children with HIV infection has been observed to be as high as 90% (Anderson & McNeilly, 1992; Belman et al., 1992). Children with HIV and AIDS experience global developmental delays, cognitive deficits, motor function abnormalities, the loss of previously acquired skills such as walking, hearing disorders, vision impairment, and microcephaly. These developmental disabilities occur within the context of difficult childrearing interactions and chronic illness (Anderson & McNeilly, 1992; Crocker & Cohen, 1990). If the number of children with AIDS continues to increase along the patterns that are predicted, HIV will become the leading infectious cause of mental retardation and developmental disability in children. The rate of HIV infection is over six times higher for Hispanic children than for European American children (U.S. Department of Health & Human Services, 1991).

Statistics suggest that American Indian children experience higher occurrences of otitis media than do non-American Indian children (Cole & Anderson, 1985). In addition, fetal alcohol syndrome (FAS) rates are higher among the American Indian populations. FAS is the cause of congenital developmental disabilities and learning disabilities.

Prematurity is the third highest cause of deafness among African American and European American children and is second highest among Asian/Pacific Americans (Nuru, 1993). Rubella is the most frequently occurring cause of deafness among Hispanic children.

## COMMUNICATION DISORDERS AMONG SCHOOL-AGE POPULATIONS

School-age children of color present with the same array of communication disorders as do European American school children. The issues that are most central to the consideration of communication disorders among culturally and linguistically diverse children are biased assessment, misdiagnosis, inappropriate educational, and clinical services.

Due to assessment procedures not being developed to accommodate cultural and linguistic diversity, it is reasonable to assume that most children of color are subjected to biased assessment. As early as the 1970s, PL 94-142 made it illegal to make determinations of communication disorders from inappropriate or discriminatory assessment procedures and instruments (Taylor, Payne & Anderson, 1987). The law stipulates that tests and evaluation materials be provided and administered in the child's native language or other mode of communication, unless it is clearly not feasible to do so. Twenty years later, the profession of speech-language pathology has not been able to completely meet the challenge of nonbiased assessment. In addressing the issue of nonbiased assessment, the ASHA has presented the following position regarding the speech-language pathologist's responsibilities (Taylor et al., 1987):

> An essential step toward making accurate assessments of communicative disorders is to distinguish between those aspects of linguistic variation that represent the diversity of the English language from those that represent speech, language, and hearing disorders. (Committee of the Status of Racial Minorities, 1983, p. 24).

Keep in mind that one of the duties of a speech-language pathologist is to distinguish normal communication development from disordered development. All normally developing children acquire and exhibit the language forms and uses of their linguistic community. A normally developing child will do so adequately; a child with communication disorders will not. The standard for assessment *must* be the communication norms of the child's linguistic community. If the speech-language pathologist has knowledge of and access to these norms, assessment can usually proceed in a nondiscriminatory manner. If the speech-language pathologist does not possess adequate knowledge of the linguistic community, nor has access to such knowledge, the assessment procedures must then be assumed to be biased. When the assessment is biased, then the diagnosis is questionable. Thus, (1) if the assessment procedures that were used were biased, and (2) if the diagnosis that results from that assessment is the presence of a communication disorder, then (3) it would not be unreasonable to question whether the diagnosis is in fact accurate.

Many sources have documented the academically related performance gaps between school children from ethnolinguistically diverse populations and European American school children. Heath (1992) studied three linguistically diverse communities, Chinese American, Mexican American, and Indo-Chinese American, to examine the influences of the home and community on the development of literacy skills among these student populations. Her premise is that there is a poor match between the kinds of language uses to which many linguistically diverse students are exposed at home and in the community and the mainstream uses of language characteristic of the school.

An important challenge exists for speech-language pathologists in delivering services to school-age children from multicultural populations. This challenge is to improve (1) the sociocultural knowledge base of the profession and (2) the practice of the professions regarding developing nondiscriminatory team-based assessment and intervention procedures. Speech-language pathologists should be collaborating proactively with classroom teachers and with English as a Second Language teachers to implement assessment and intervention.

Nuru (1993) provides interesting multicultural perspectives regarding hearing disorders. She documents that while the total number of deaf and hard-of-hearing children is decreasing in this country, the proportion of children of color among the deaf is increasing. To illustrate, in 1980 children of color represented 22.5% of hearing impaired children and 36.6% in 1990. The most significant increase is among Hispanic children, however, increases are seen among all non-European American ethnic groups.

Nuru (1993) has also discovered multicultural variation in terms of etiologies of hearing impairment. Meningitis and heredity are primary causes of hearing loss across all populations; however, meningitis disproportionately affects African American and American Indian children. Heredity disproportionately affects European American, Hispanic, and American Indians. Meningitis is the primary cause of deafness among American Indians (16.2%) and African Americans (14%), almost doubling the prevalence among European American (8.8%) and Hispanic (6.8%), and, almost quadrupling the occurrence among Asian/Pacific Americans (4%).

## COMMUNICATION DISORDERS AMONG ADULT POPULATIONS

Diabetes is 33% more common among African Americans than among European Americans. The highest rates are among African American women (U.S. Department of Health & Human Services, 1991). Among the many complications of diabetes is hearing loss (Carter, 1984).

Hispanics experience tremendous variety in their profile because of the different subgroupings based on countries of origin. For example, whereas Mexican Americans experience low rates of cerebrovascular disease, a major cause of strokes, stroke rates among Puerto Ricans are high. Cerebrovascular accident (CVA) causes strokes, and depending on the locus of the cerebral lesion, aphasia may occur. Aphasia refers to the loss of language due to trauma to the brain. African Americans also have a high prevalence of hypertension, which would suggest that aphasia would be a communication disorder many Hispanic and African American adults would experience as a consequence of strokes. Peters-Johnson and Taylor (1986) note that given the tendency toward hypertension among various ethnic groups, it is "rather incredible to note the paucity of research on aphasia" (p. 172).

Wallace and Freeman (1991) administered a clinical survey to obtain information about general client characteristics for adults with neurological impairment from multicultural populations and about the clinical services provided to them. Thirty programs were surveyed and the results revealed low numbers of adults are serviced. Another finding was that these individuals received services for only a short period of time, for 1–2 months. The one word that resonates from this study is *underutilization*—underutilization of services. There is tremendous need for speech, language, and hearing facilities to improve their marketing efforts in order to improve service delivery to people of color who are experiencing communication disorders due to neurological impairment.

AIDS is quite a pervasive disease in many cities and towns of the United States, and adults of color have an alarmingly high incidence of the disease. In 1985 African Americans comprised 12% of the nation's population; however, during that year African Americans represented 27% of diagnosed AIDS cases (Wallace, 1993). Wallace reports that in 1988 the Centers for Disease Control estimated that approximately 57% of all AIDS cases were European Americans, 26% were African Americans, 15% were Hispanic Americans, 1% were Asian/Pacific Americans, and less than 1% were Native Americans. The relationship between AIDS and communication disorders is that during the later stages of the disease, neurophychological deficits often develop, deficits which impair the individual's communication abilities. For example, memory loss, motor speech impairment, dysphagia, reduced concentration, and reduced performance on cognitive tasks frequently are observed among patients with AIDS, and these deficits reduce one's ability to produce and process communication effectively.

Regarding hearing disorders, sickle cell anemia is linked to hearing loss. Sickle cell anemia primarily affects people of African descent. Studies of adults with sickle cell anemic reveal that many present with sensorineural hearing loss (Buchanan, Moore, & Counter, 1993). These authors also indicate that African Americans show less permanent losses in hearing levels than European Americans when subjected to excessive noise exposure. Moreover, Meniere disease, a complex syndrome of hearing disorder consisting of vertigo, hearing loss, and tinnitus, shows multicultural variation. The prevalence rate of Meniere disease is estimated as being 1:2500 among European American populations and 1:25,000 among Asian populations (Buchanan et al., 1993).

## CONCLUSIONS

The aim of this chapter has been to present introductory information on communication disorders among multicultural populations. Admittedly, in-depth discussions have not been provided; however, it is clear that much more research needs to be conducted. The notion of cultural diversity in the presence of communication disorders is relatively new. There are many questions to be asked and many topics to be explored. As students in the field of communication sciences and disorders, begin to investigate this topic yourself. Best practices in speech-language pathology and in audiology come from research— field research and empirical investigation. Continued progress in the area of multicultural perspectives in communication disorders requires the attention of future professionals. By writing this text, we have attempted to both inform and to motivate. The professions of audiology and speech-language pathology need to attract committed, inquisitive, and creative students who are interested in advancing knowledge and in addressing the communication needs of the underserved.

# 10

# Profiles of Audiologists and Speech-Language Pathologists Representing Diverse Cultural and Linguistic Groups

## RHONDA FRIEDLANDER
Speech-Language Pathologist
*American Indian*

To her people, the Ktunaxa Nation, Rhonda Friedlander is known as Ukup G̠ǂata Paǂki—One-Claw-From-a-Grizzly-Bear-Woman. It's a powerful name by Ktunaxa standards. The grizzly bear is a revered protector of the people.

Friedlander holds the distinction of being the first certified speech-language pathologist of the Kootenai tribe. Not so long ago, her greatest ambition was to become a college sophomore.

"I was proud to make it past my freshman year. The move from reservation to college campus was traumatic. I was terribly homesick. You have to understand how close ties are among tribal members." Just how close is illustrated by this fact: There is no Kootenai word for cousin. "Our tribe is our family. Every woman younger than me is my *kanana*, younger sister. Every woman older is my *katsu*. Anything that happens is as if it happened to my blood sister."

Not only did Friedlander graduate from college (she received her BS from Gonazaga University, Spokane, Washington), she went on to receive her MS from Eastern Washington University, Cheney. Now she is the speech-language pathologist for the Confederated Salish and

Kootenal Tribes of the Flathead Reservation, Montana. In addition to providing services to four Head Start centers, two day-care centers, two health clinics, a tribal high school, and a convalescent center, she also conducts regular home visits. Friedlander is, in effect, her own program administrator and head clinician.

And this from a woman who was told she would never graduate from high school. "There was lots of discrimination when I was growing up on the reservation."

What gave her the will to persist?

"I always felt powerful and strong—like my name," says Friedlander. "I also knew from the time I was a child that I wanted to help my people." Her mother and grandmother told her one way to do that was to get a White man's education.

Friedlander's special interests are in adapting standardized testing materials for Native American relevancy and in preventing otitis media and fetal alcohol syndrome (FAS) in Native American populations.

Friedlander and the late Lynn Larrigan, formerly of Washington State University, developed a paraprofessional training program for the Bureau of Indian Affairs. This program trains other Native Americans to provide speech and language services and hearing screenings on their own reservations.

---

Reprinted from *ASHA*, May, 1992, 21, with permission.

---

## SYLVIA ALLEN
Audiologist
*European American*

While working as a registered nurse at an eye, ear, nose, and throat (ENT) hospital, I became interested in the services the speech-languages provided to the laryngectomized patients. I took an introductory course in speech and hearing at the local university, became interested in audiology, and recognized a unique opportunity to combine my ENT nursing experience with a career in audiology.

Part-time and private duty ENT nursing jobs helped to pay my tuition through a master's degree program in audiology, allowing me to then obtain ASHA certification and clinical audiology positions at major medical centers—including the hospital where I had been an ENT nurse.

Work with hearing researchers at Walter Reed Army Medical Center in Washington, DC, led me to complete a Ph.D. program at Vanderbilt University in Nashville, TN, and, most recently, an NIH-sponsored postdoctoral fellowship in auditory anatomy and physiology at the Kresge Hearing Research Laboratory at Louisiana State University in New Orleans. I have had staff and supervisory positions in audiology, served on the faculty of speech and hearing departments, and am currently teaching graduate courses in electrophysiology.

I have completed auditory research on brain anatomy, pathology, histology, and evoked potentials. Currently, I am doing intraoperative monitoring of evoked potentials recorded from cranial and spinal nerves during brain and spinal surgery. I also collect and interpret evoked potential data on babies in intensive care nurseries providing important hearing and neurodiagnostic data for their care.

> Reprinted from Autobiographical Sketches: ASHA Members Who Previously Worked or Majored in Another Field, in Chabon, S.S., Cole, P.A., Culatta, R.A., Lorendo, L.C., & Terry, S.E. (Eds.), Speech-Language Pathology and Audiology Student Recruitment Manual, Rockville, American Speech-Language-Hearing Association, 1990, with permission.

## LI-RONG LILLY CHENG
Speech-Language Pathologist
*Asian American*

When I first came to the US as a foreign-born international student, my goal was to pursue the field of linguistics with a focus on teaching English as a foreign language. After two years of study, I found myself struggling with the subject matter and feeling depressed that I did not possess the "native speaker's intuition." I was further struck by the complexity of the English language, its form, content, and function. I also realized that language is embedded in culture and that sociolinguistics and metalinguistic skills do not come from reading books but from experience and interaction with others.

One day, I went to the speech clinic on campus to seek some advice and discovered the field of communication disorders. Since that winter morning in 1970, I have devoted my time and energy to understand this challenging, rewarding, and dynamic field. I am currently the assistant dean for Student Affairs and International Development in the College of Health and Human Services, a faculty member of the Department of Communicative Disorders and the coordinator for the Bilingual/Multicultural Certificate program at San Diego State University.

My research interests include topics dealing with working with the ever-growing bilingual/multicultural diverse populations in this nation, and I have written on these topics. In addition, I have coordinated many conferences and symposia on the topics of communication disorders and facilitated faculty exchanges between San Diego State University and academic institutions in the Pacific Rim. I contribute what little I know about the difficulties of being a nonnative speaker and a person from a totally different culture.

I love this field, and I am sure you will also.

> Reprinted from: Autobiographical Sketches: ASHA Members Who Previously Worked or Majored in Another Field, in Chabon, S.S., Cole, P.A., Culatta, R.A., Lorendo, L.C., & Terry, S.E. (Eds.), Speech-Language Pathology and Audiology Student Recruitment Manual, Rockville, American Speech-Language-Hearing Association, 1990, with permission.

## LORRAINE T. COLE
Speech-Language Pathologist
*African American*

After working for a few years as a certified speech-language pathologist in various settings, I found myself gravitating toward professional conferences and publications in the field of linguistics. I ultimately gave in to this "inner voice." I enrolled in a second master's degree program in applied linguistics while I continued as a speech-language pathologist.

I was giving serious consideration to leaving the profession of speech-language pathology to pursue a doctorate in linguistics when I met Dr. Roy Koenigsknecht. At the time, he headed the speech-language pathology program at Northwestern University and he convinced me that I could "have it both ways." That is, I could conduct applied linguistics research within the field of communicative disorders. And, I have done exactly that!

I earned a Ph.D. in speech-language pathology from Northwestern University and have been awarded research fellowships from the Ford and Rockefeller Foundations to conduct applied linguistics research. I have further expanded my interests in linguistics to include communication disorders among linguistically and culturally diverse populations. [Dr. Cole served as] director of Minority Concerns in the National Office of the American Speech-Language-Hearing Association.

> Reprinted from Autobiographical Sketches: ASHA Members Who Previously Worked or Majored in Another Field, in Chabon, S.S., Cole, P.A., Culatta, R.A., Lorendo, L.C., & Terry, S.E. (Eds.), Speech-Language Pathology and Audiology Student Recruitment Manual, Rockville, American Speech-Language-Hearing Association, 1990, with permission.

## TERESITA FOSTER
Speech-Language Pathologist
*Peruvian*

I am a Bi-lingual Speech-Language Pathologist. I obtained my bachelor's degree in 1971 from the National Teacher's College in Peru; I received my Master of Science degree in Speech-Language Pathology in 1987 from the University of the District of Columbia; and I was awarded the Certificate of Clinical Competence in Speech-Language Pathology (CCC-SP) in 1988.

I also received certification as a Bi-lingual/Bi-cultural Assessment Specialist from the George Washington University in 1989. In addition, I have taken several courses in linguistics at Georgetown University. I now am beginning the doctoral program in Communication Disorders at Howard University as a CHMM-OSERS Fellow.

Although my interests in communication disorders began while working with normal and learning disabled children in Peru, these interests in communication disorders and bilingualism became my principal professional and personal goals in 1983 after I moved to the United States to begin married life. Because I could not speak English fluently, I found that many people assumed that I had a communication problem or deficit. This, plus my prior work experience, made me decide that my professional life interests should be study and research on the identification of communication disorders and culturally sensitive ways to accurately differentiate true communication disorders from dialectal variations among English native speakers, and from the stages that child and adult Spanish native speakers go through as they acquire English as a second language. I currently work as a Bi-lingual Speech-Language Pathologist in the District of Columbia Public School system.

*Source:* Written for this text by Teresita Foster.

## ERNEST J. MOORE
Audiologist
*African American*

I was a student majoring in radio and television broadcasting at Tennessee State University (TSU) in Nashville, TN. A friend told me about her son who was hard-of-hearing, and how she had been trying to enroll him in a school for children with hearing impairments. She indicated that she had taken him to the Central Institute for the Deaf in St. Louis where hearing tests had been performed by an audiologist.

The manner in which she described the hearing tests given to her son caught my interest.

Shortly thereafter, I decided to obtain more information about audiological testing. I visited the nearby Bill Wilkerson Speech and Hearing Clinic at Vanderbilt University. There I met an audiologist, who showed me what he did to test hearing. Since the audiological equipment was somewhat similar to radio and television broadcasting equipment, I found my interest piqued.

The next step was to discuss with my college department chairperson how I might enter the field. At his suggestion, I took courses in speech and audiological sciences and later switched my major from radio and television to audiology and speech sciences. All of the audiology courses were taught by various staff from Vanderbilt University who taught at TSU in the evenings. It just so happens that the instructors from Vanderbilt were all Euro-Americans—my classmates were all African Americans. At that time, African Americans were not permitted to enroll in courses in predominantly white universities.

After receiving my undergraduate and master's degrees in audiology, I developed a strong interest in research and academic teaching. I was encouraged by Dr. Darrell Rose to enroll in a doctoral program in audiology. After receiving my doctorate, I held research, teaching, and clinical positions at Emerson College, Harvard University Health Services, Memphis State University, and an administrative post at the National Institutes of Health. For six years, I served as professor and chairperson, Department of Audiology and Speech Sciences at Michigan State University (MSU). In 1983, I edited the first textbook on auditory brain-stem evoked potentials. Presently I am professor of Audiology at MSU where I continue to conduct research on various aspects of the auditory system.

---

Reprinted from Autobiographical Sketches: ASHA Members Who Previously Worked or Majored in Another Field, in Chabon, S.S., Cole, P.A., Culatta, R.A., Lorendo, L.C., & Terry, S.E. (Eds.), Speech-Language Pathology and Audiology Student Recruitment Manual, Rockville, American Speech-Language-Hearing Association, 1990, with permission.

---

## MARK YLVISAKER
Speech-Language Pathologist
*European American*

When I was a junior in high school, I became interested in philosophy by reading philosophy of science books in conjunction with my physics course. I continued this interest through college, graduated with the highest honors in philosophy, German, and English literature, and attended graduate school on a Woodrow Wilson Fellowship. Subsequently, I taught philosophy for four years.

I decided to change careers during a year in Heidelberg, Germany, working on my Ph.D. dissertation in philosophy. The attractions of speech-language pathology for me were (a) I wanted a clinically engaging career that offered a wide variety of possibilities; (b) I wanted a career in which I could easily combine clinical work, research, and teaching; (c) I wanted a career in which I could make a contribution; and, (d) I did not want to spend an extraordinary amount of time retraining for a new career.

I am currently program director of an inpatient head injury rehabilitation program. In this capacity, I oversee the clinical program and all of the rehabilitation professionals. To say that my career in speech-language pathology has been engaging would be a sizeable understatement. I even think that I have made a small contribution, having published two books and more than 30 journal articles and book chapters on head injury rehabilitation.

---

Reprinted from Autobiographical Sketches: ASHA Members Who Previously Worked or Majored in Another Field, in Chabon, S.S., Cole, P.A., Culatta, R.A., Lorendo, L.C., & Terry, S.E. (Eds.), Speech-Language Pathology and Audiology Student Recruitment Manual, Rockville, American Speech-Language-Hearing Association, 1990, with permission.

# References

Abbas, A. Y. (1992). Cleft lip and palate in Tehran. *The Cleft Palate-Craniofacial Journal, 29,* 15.

Altemus, L. A. (1966). The incidence of cleft lip and cleft palate among North American Negroes. *Cleft Palate Journal, 3,* 357.

Anderson, N. B., & Battle, D. (1993). Cultural diversity in the development of language. In D. Battle (Ed.), *Communication disorders in multicultural populations* (pp. 158-182). Boston: Andover Medical Publishers.

Anderson, N. B., & Lee-Wilkerson, D. L. (1993). Reaching multicultural populations. *ASHA, 35,* 43-44, 51.

Anderson, N. B., & McNeilly, L. G. (1992). Meeting the needs of special populations. In M. Bender & C. A. Baglin (Eds.), *Infants and toddlers: A resource guide for practitioners* (pp. 49-68). San Diego: Singular Publishing Group.

ASHA. (1969a). Bowden appointed special assistant for urban affairs. *ASHA, 11*(9), 398-399.

ASHA. (1969b). Social and political involvement of the American Speech and Hearing Association. *ASHA, 11*(5), 216-217.

ASHA. (1970). Legislative council report. *ASHA, 12,* 186-199.

ASHA. (1971a). Bowden leaves national office. *ASHA, 10,* 622.

ASHA. (1971b). Legislative council report. *ASHA, 13,* 136.

ASHA. (1971c). Legislative council report. *ASHA, 13,* 275.

ASHA. (1971d). Special reports. *ASHA, 13,* 275.

ASHA. (1972). Special tribute paid to Jack Bangs. *ASHA, 14,* 26.

ASHA. (1973a). ASHA appoints John B. Joyner to head urban, ethnic affairs. *ASHA, 15,* 361.

ASHA. (1973b). Legislative council report. *ASHA, 15,* 131.

ASHA. (1983). Legislative council report. *ASHA, 25,* 173.

ASHA. (1985). ASHA interviews Lorraine Cole. *ASHA, 27,* 7-10.

ASHA. (1991). Multicultural action agenda 2000. *ASHA, 33,* 39-41.

ASHA. (1993). Legislative council report. *ASHA, 35,* 29-36.

Battle, D. E. (1993). *Communication disorders in multicultural populations.* Boston: Andover Medical Publishers.

Bebout, L., & Bradford, A. (1992). Crosscultural attitudes toward speech disorders. *Brain and Language, 41,* 437-445.

Belman, A. L., Diamond, G., Dickson, D., Horoupian, D., Llena, J., Langos, G., & Rubinstein, A. (1992). Pediatric acquired immunodeficiency syndrome: Neurological syndromes. *American Journal of Disordered Children, 142,* 29-35.

Bloom, L., & Lahey, M. (1978). *Language development and language disorders.* New York: John Wiley & Sons.

Bountress, N. (1987). The Ann Arbor decision in retrospect. *ASHA, 29*(9), 55-57.

Brewer, J. M. (1968). *American Negro folklore.* Chicago: Quadrangle Books.

Brown, S. (1953). Negro folk expression: Spirituals, seculars, ballads and work songs. *Phylon, 14,* 50-60.

Buchanan, L. H., Moore, E. J., & Counter, S. A. (1993). Hearing disorders and auditory assessment. In D. Battle (Ed.), *Communication disorders in multicultural populations* (pp. 256-279). Boston: Andover Medical Publishers.

Campbell, L. (1985). *Training needs of speech-language pathologists.* Doctoral dissertation, Howard University, Washington, DC.

Carter, R. (1984, April). *Hearing loss and diabetes.* Paper presented at the annual national convention of the National Black Association for Speech, Language and Hearing, Detroit, Michigan.

Chabon, S. S., Cole, P. T., Culatta, R. A., Lorendo, L. C., & Terry, S. E. (Eds.), (1990). *Speech-language pathology and audiology student recruitment manual.* Rockville, MD: American Speech-Language-Hearing Association.

Char, E. L. (1981). The Chinese American. In A. L. Clark (Ed.), *Culture and childrearing.* Philadelphia: F.A. Davis Company.

Cheng, L. (1989). Service delivery to Asian/Pacific LEP children: A crosscultural framework. *Topics in Language Disorders, 9,* 1-14.

Chinn, P. C., & Hughes, S. (1987). Representation of minority students in special education classes. *Remedial and Special Education, 8*(4), 41-46.

Cole, L. T. (1980). Blacks with orofacial clefts: The state of the dilemma. *ASHA, 22,* 557-560.

Cole, L. T. (1987). *Minority brain drain in human communication sciences and disorders.* Unpublished material, ED 187178.

Cole, L. T. (1989). E pluribus pluribus: Multicultural imperatives and the 1990's and beyond. *ASHA, 31,* 65-70.

Cole, L. T. (in press). Cleft palate: A sample course syllabus on orofacial anomalies. In Cole, L. & V. Deal (Eds.), *Communication disorders in multicultural populations.* Rockville, MD: American Speech-Language-Hearing Association.

Cole, L., & Anderson, N. B. (1985). The economicqally disadvantaged. In L. Cole (Ed.), *National colloquium on underserved populations,* Rockville, MD: American Speech-Language-Hearing Association.

Cole, L., & Massey, A. (1985). Minority student enrollment in higher education institutions with communicative disorders programs. *ASHA, 27*(6), 33-37.

Committee on Status of Racial Minorities (1983). *Clinical management of communicatively handicapped minority language population, ASHA, 27,* 6-10.

Council of Graduate Programs in Communication Sciences and Disorders. (1984). *1983-84 National Survey.* Minneapolis, MN.

Council of Graduate Programs in Communication Sciences and Disorders. (1985). *1984-85 National Survey.* Minneapolis, MN.

Council of Graduate Programs in Communication Sciences and Disorders. (1986). *1985-86 National Survey.* Minneapolis, MN.

Council of Graduate Programs in Communication Sciences and Disorders. (1991). *1990-91 National Survey.* Minneapolis, MN.

Courlander, H. (1963). *Negro folk music, USA.* New York: Columbia University Press.

Crocker, A. C., & Cohen, H. J. (1990). *Guidelines on developmental services for children and adults with HIV infection.* Silver Spring, MD: American Association of University Affiliated Programs.

Cummins, J. (1992). Language proficiency, bilingualism, and academic achievement. In P. A. Richard-Amato & M. A. Snow (Eds.), *The multicultural classroom* (pp. 16-26). White Plains, NY: Longman.

Dalby, D. (1971). Black through White: Patterns of communication in Africa and the New World. In W. Wolfram & N. Clarke (Eds.), *Black-White speech relationships.* Washington, DC: Center for Applied Linguistics.

Davis, H. (1972, July 26). Memorandum sent to A. Zaner.

Davis, H., & Silverman, S. R. (1978). *Hearing and deafness.* New York: Holt, Rinehart, and Winston.

Dillard, J. L. (1972). *Black English: Its history and usage in the United States.* New York: Random House.

Dillard, J. M. (1983). *Multicultural counseling.* Chicago: Nelson-Hall.

Dunn, L. (1968). Special education for the mildly retarded: Is much of it justifiable? *Exceptional Children, 7,* 5-24.

Educational Testing Service. (1990, October). *Analyses of Educational Testing Service data.* Princeton, NJ: Author.

Ehling, M. B. (1981). The Mexican American. In A. L. Clark (Ed.), *Culture and childrearing.* Philadelphia: F.A. Davis Company.

Farris, C. E., & Farris, L. J. (1981). The American Indian. In A. L. Clark (Ed.), *Culture and childrearing.* Philadelphia: F.A. Davis Company.

First Hispanic Caucus Membership Forum. (1993). *Hispanic Caucus for Speech-Language Pathologists and Audiologists Newsletter, 1*(1), 4.

Fisher, M. M. (1953). *Negro slave songs in the United States.* Ithaca, NY: Cornell University Press.

Ford, S. L. (1983). *A glimpse of the National Black Association of Speech, Language and Hearing.* Unpublished manuscript.

Garrett, R. (1966). African survivals in American culture. *Journal of Negro History, 51,* 239-245.

Gee, J. P. (1985). The narrativization of experience in the oral style. *Journal of Education, 167,* 9-35.

Gollnick, D. M., & Chinn, P. C. (1990). *Multicultural education in a pluralistic society.* Columbus, OH: Merrill Publishing Co.

Greathouse, B., & Miller, V. G. (1981). The Black American. In A. L. Clark (Ed.), *Culture and childrearing.* Philadelphia: F.A. Davis Company.

Hanson, M. J., Lynch, E. W., & Wayman, K. I. (1990). Honoring the cultural diversity of families when gathering data. *Topics in Early Childhood Special Education, 10,* 112-131.

Heath, S. B. (1992). Sociocultural contexts of language development: Implications for the classroom. In P. A. Richard-Amato & M. A. Snow (Ed.), *The multicultural classroom* (pp. 102-125). White Plains, NY: Longman.

Heath, S. B. (1982). What no bedtime story means: Narrative skills at home and school. *Language and Society, 11,* 49-76.

Herskovits, M. (1941). *The myth of the Negro past.* New York: Harper & Brothers.

Hook, E. & Harlap, S. (1979). Differences in maternal agespecific rates of Down syndrome between Jews of European origin and of North African or Asian origin. *Teratology, 20,* 243-248.

Iglesias, A., & Anderson, N. B. (1993). Dialectal variations. In J. Bernthall & N. Bankson (Eds.), *Articulation and phonological disorders* (pp. 147-161). Englewood Cliffs, NJ: Prentice-Hall.

Jeter, I. K. (1977). *American Speech and Hearing Association minority education workshop proceedings.* Rockville, MD: American Speech and Hearing Association.

Kayser, H. (1993). More minority presenters needed. *Hispanic Caucus for Speech-Language Pathologists and Audiologists Newsletter, 1(1),* 4.

Lau vs. Nichols, 411 U.S. 563 (1974).

Leith, W., & Mims, H. A. (1975). Cultural influences in the development and treatment of stuttering: A preliminary report on the black stutterer. *Journal of Speech and Hearing Research, 40,* 459-466.

Luterman, D. M. (1991). *Counseling the communicatively disordered and their families.* Austin, TX: Pro-Ed.

Mayfield, S. (1984, April). *Excess lead absorption and communication disorders in black children.* Paper presented at the annual convention of the National Black Association on Speech, Language and Hearing, Detroit, MI.

Mercer, J. (1973). *Labeling the mentally retarded.* Los Angeles: University of California Press.

Millard, D., & McNeill, K. A. (1965). The incidence of cleft lip and palate in Jamaica. *The Cleft Palate Journal, 2,* 384-388.

Myrianthopoulous, N. C., & Chung, C. S. (1974). Congenital malformations in singletons: Epidemiologic survey. *Report from the collaborative perinatal project.* New York: Medical Book Corp.

NBASLH. (1992). *Fourteenth Annual convention luncheon program.*

NBASLH. (1979, October). *Notes.*

Nuru, N. (1993). Multicultural aspects of deafness. In D. Battle (Ed.), *Communication disorders in multicultural populations* (pp. 287-302). Boston: Andover Medical Publishers.

PDR Steering Committee. (1971). Letter addressed to members of ASHA.

Payne, J., & Stockman, I. (1979). Sickle cell disease recommendations for research and clinical services in speech pathology and audiology. *Journal of Allied Health, 2*(3), 257-264.

Payne, K. T., Anderson, N. B., & Cole, P. (1988). *NESPA project: Plenary session.* Unpublished material.

Peters-Johnson, C. A. & Taylor, O. L. (1986). Speech, language and hearing disorders in Black populations. In O. L. Taylor (Ed.), *Nature of communication disorders in culturally and linguistically diverse populations* (pp. 157-179). San Diego: College-Hill Press.

Ramirez, B. (1988). Culturally and linguistically diverse children, *Teaching Exceptional Children, 45,* 45-81.

Royster, L. H., Driscoll, D. P., Thomas, W. G., & Royster, J. D. (1980). Age effect hearing levels for black non-industrial noise exposed population (NINEP) *American Industrial Hygiene Association Journal, 41,* 113-119.

Schenerle, J. (1992). *Counseling in speech-language pathology and audiology.* New York: Macmillan Publishing Company.

Schoendorf, K. C., Hogue, C. J. R., Kleinman, J. C., & Rowley, D. (1992). Mortality among infants of black as compared with white college-educated parents. *The New England Journal of Medicine, 326,* 1522-1526.

Scott, D. M. (in press). Hearing disorders in multicultural populations. In L. Cole & V. Deal (Eds.), *Communication disorders in multicultural populations.* Rockville, MD: American Speech-Language-Hearing Association.

Screen, R. M., & Taylor, H. (1972). Relevancy of speech and hearing facilities to the Black community. *Language, Speech and Hearing Services in the Schools, 3,* 56-61.

Shames, G. H. (1989). Stuttering: An RFP for a cultural perspective. *Journal of Fluency Disorders, 14,* 67-77.

Smith, T. (1992). Multicultural focus groups. *ASHA, 34,* 53.

Stewart, C. H. (1971, October 27). Letter to ASHA Black Caucus.

Stewart, W. (1971). Sociolinguistic factors in the history of American Negro dialects. In W. Wolfram & N. Clarke (Eds.), *Black-White speech relationships,* Washington, DC: Center for Applied Linguistics.

Stockman I. J. (1986). Language acquisition in culturally diverse populations: The black child as a case study. In O. L. Taylor (Ed.), *Nature of communication disorders in culturally and linguistically diverse populations* (pp. 117-155). San Diego, College-Hill Press.

Stockman, I. J., Vaughn-Cooke, F. B., & Wolfram W. (1982). *A developmental study of Black English—Phase I.* Washington, DC: Center for Applied Linguistics.

Stockman, I. J., & Vaughn-Cooke, F. (1992). Lexical elaboration in children's locative action expressions. *Child Development, 63,* 1104-1125.

Stuckey, S. (1968). Through the prism of folklore: The black ethos in slavery. *Massachusetts Review, 9,* 417-437.

Sue, D. W., & Sue, D. (1990). *Counseling the culturally different.* New York: John Wiley & Sons.

Tanaka, T. (1972). A clinical, genetic, and epidemiologic study on cleft lip and/or palate. *Japanese Journal of Human Genetics, 16,* 278.

Taylor, J. (1992). *Speech-language pathology services in the public schools.* Boston: Allyn & Bacon.

Taylor, O. L. (in press). Clinical practice as a social occasion. In L. Cole & V. Deal (Eds.), *Communication disorders in multicultural populations.* Rockville, MD: American Speech-Language-Hearing Association.

Taylor, O. L., Payne, K. T., & Anderson, N. B. (1987). Distinguishing between communication disorders and communication differences. *Seminars in Speech and Language, 8,* 415-427.

Taylor, O. L., Stroud, R. V., Hurst, C. G., Moore, E. J., & Williams, R. (1969). Philosophies and goals of the ASHA black caucus. *ASHA, 11,* 221-225.

Thomas, G. E. (1983). The deficit, difference and bicultural theories of black dialect and nonstandard English. *The Urban Review, 15,* 107-118.

Tretsven, V. E. (1963). Incidence of cleft lip and palate in Montana Indians. *Journal of Speech and Hearing Disorders, 7,* 52.

Tsutsui, H. (1951). Study on the etiology of clefts of the lip and the palate: Clinico-statistical observations (in Japanese). *Journal of Dentists (Japan), 8,* 3.

Valentine, C. A. (1971). Deficit, difference and bicultural models of Afro-American behavior. *Harvard Educational Review, 41,* 137-157.

U.S. Department of Health & Human Services. (1991). *Healthy people 2000.* (Pub. No. PHS 9150213). Washington, DC: Author.

Vanderas, A. P. (1987). Incidence of cleft lip and cleft palate among races: A review. *The Cleft Palate Journal, 24,* 216-225.

Van Riper, C. (1971). *The nature of stuttering.* Englewood Cliffs, NJ: Prentice-Hall.

Vaughn-Cooke, F. B. (1983). Improving langage assessment in minority children. *ASHA, 25*(9), 29-33.

Wallace, G. L. (1993). Adult neurogenic disorders. In D. Battle (Ed.), *Communication disorders in multicultural populations* (pp. 239-249). Boston: Andover Medical Publishers.

Wallace, G. L., & Freeman, S. B. (1991). Adults with neurological impairments from multicultural populations. *ASHA, 33* (June/July), 58-60.

Webster, E. J. (1977). *Counseling with parents of handicapped children.* New York: Grune & Stratton.

# Index

African Americans. *See also* Black Caucus; National Black Association for Speech, Language and Hearing (NBASLH)
AIDS, 106
audiology, 113-114
childrearing practices, 86-88
children
    discourse development, 75-76
    mild mental retardation classification, 78
cleft palate, 98
deafness, 104
Down syndrome, 101, 102
HIV-positive, 10, 103
lead blood levels high, 10
low birth weight, 9-10, 103
meningitis, 105
otitis media, 9
and perception, 82
presbycusis, 9
professional enrollment, 20, 21
sickle cell anemia, 9, 107
speech/hearing facility relevancy, 83
as speech-language pathology (SLP)/audiology students, 18-20
storytelling traditions, 70-71
stuttering, 100-101
test norms, 11
Africanisms, 69-71
AIDS, 106-107. *See* HIV-positive
African Americans, 106
American English. *See* Standard American English

American Indian Professional Training Program, University of Arizona, 47
American Indians, 109-110. *See also* Native American Caucus of the ASHA; Native Americans
fetal alcohol syndrome (FAS), 103, 110
meningitis, 105
National Examinations in Speech-Language Pathology and Audiology (NESPA), 22
otitis media, 9, 103, 110
Professional Training Program, University of Arizona, 47
speech-language pathology (SLP), 109-110
as speech-language pathology (SLP)/audiology students, 18-20
test norms, 12
American Speech-Language-Hearing Association (ASHA). *See also* Black Caucus; National Black Association for Speech, Language and Hearing (NBASLH)
Committee on the Status of Racial Minorities, 53
defined, 3
dialectal differences statement, 93-94
Institute on Teaching Cultural Diversity, vii
minority-related resolutions, Legislative Council, 57-64
Office of Multicultural Affairs, x, 23, 82-83

Asian Americans. *See also* Chinese
Americans
National Examinations in Speech-
Language Pathology and
Audiology (NESPA), 22
 otitis media, 9
 speech-language pathology (SLP),
111-112
 as speech-language pathology
(SLP)/audiology students,
18-20
 test norms, 12, 105
Asians/Pacific Islanders
 cleft palate, 98-99
 deafness, 104
 Down syndrome, 101, 102
 stuttering, 100-101
Assessment. *See* Testing
At-risk births, 8-9
Audiology
 African Americans, 113-114
 counseling, multicultural, 81-94
 European Americans, 110-111
 eye, ear nose, and throat (ENT)
nursing, 110
 multicultural professionals, 17-29
 professional barriers, 20-24
 Spanish speaking, 84-85

Basic interpersonal communicative
skills (BICS), 79
Bidialectualism, 72
Bilingual Education Act of 1976, 95
Black Caucus. *See also* African
Americans
 American Speech-Language-
Hearing Association (ASHA)
  Executive Associate Secretary
for African American
Affairs, 34
 founding, 31-32
 Resolution 42, 35-37, 40-41
 Special Assistant for Urban
Affairs, 37-39
Black English. *See* Black English
Vernacular
Black English Vernacular, 55-56. *See
also* Dialects

Africanisms, 69-71
AfroEnglish, 66-67
AfroFrench, 67
AfroSpanish, 67
bidialectualism, 72
Gullah dialect, 69-70
phonology/syntax, 71-72
pidgin, early, 69
slavery and language
development, 67-72
Bureau of Indian Affairs,
paraprofessional training, 110

Caucasians. *See also* European
Americans; White Americans
cleft palate, 97-98
Cerebral palsy, 8, 9, 103
Cerebrovascular accident (CVA), 106
Certificate of Clinical Competence
(CCC), 113
Certificate of Clinical Competence
(CCC), sociolinguistics, 34-35
Certification, professional, 21-22
Childrearing practices, 86-94
Children
 African Americans, 73-76
  mild mental retardation
classification, 78
 at-risk births, 8
 childrearing practices, 86-94
 low birth weight, 8-10
 native Americans, 46-47
 preschool, 102-104
 school-age, 104-105
 Spanish speaking, 77, 78, 84-85
 special education placement, 80
Chinese Americans. *See also* Asian
Americans
 childrearing practices, 88-91
Cleft palate, 97-99
Clinical Fellowship Year (CFY), 21, 23
 Native American Caucus of the
ASHA, 46
Clinical practice
 guilt/paternalism, 85
 language sensitivity, 84
 and Native American children,
46-47

Clinical practice (continued)
  and socioeconomics, 13
  stereotype countermeasures, 85-86
Cognitive/academic language
  proficiency (CALP), 79
Communication disorders
  adult, 106-107
  AIDS, 106-107
  cleft palate, 97-99
  Meniere disease, 107
  overdiagnosis, 95-96
  preschool, 102-104
  school-age, 104-105
  stuttering, 100-101
  underdiagnosis, 95-96
Counseling, perception, role of, 81-83

Deafness, 104, 105. *See also* Hearing
  impairment
Demographics, people of color
  population growth, 17-18
Diabetes, 106
Dialects, 53-54. *See also* Black English
  Vernacular
  Africanisms, 69-71
  Ann Arbor Decision (Martin
    Luther King Junior
    Elementary School v. Ann
    Arbor School District), 55-56
  bidialectualism, 72
  Gullah, 69-70
  Lau v. Nichols, 54-55
  sociolinguistics, 65-66
  speech-language pathology (SLP)
    guidelines, 77
Disability. *See* PL 94-142, the
  Education for All
  Handicapped Children Act
  (EHA), PL 99-457, Individuals
  with Disabilities Education
  Act (IDEA)
Disorders, communication. *See*
  Communication disorders
Down syndrome, 101-102

Ebonics. *See* Black English Vernacular
Educational programming, 78-80

EHA. *See* PL 94-142, the Education
  for All Handicapped Children
  Act (EHA)
European Americans. *See also*
  Caucasians; White Americans
  audiology, 110-111
  speech-language pathology (SLP),
    114-115
European trade languages, 69

Fetal alcohol syndrome (FAS)
  American Indians, 110
Fetal alcohol syndrome (FAS),
  American Indians, 103

Handicapped. *See* PL 94-142, the
  Education for All Handi-
  capped Children Act (EHA),
  PL 99-457, Individuals with
  Disabilities Education Act
  (IDEA)
Health paradigms, multicultural,
  12-13
Hearing impairment, 105. *See also*
  Deafness
  and diabetes, 106
Hearing/speech facility relevancy,
  83
Hispanic Caucus of the ASHA
  founding, 47-48
  goals, 48-49
Hispanics. *See also* Mexican
  Americans; Puerto Ricans;
  Spanish-speaking
  and audiology, 84-85
  deafness, 104
  Down syndrome, 101
  Hearing impairment, 105
  HIV-positive, 103
  Lead blood levels high, 10
  rubella, 104
  as speech-language pathology
    (SLP)/audiology students,
    18-20
HIV-positive, 8. *See* AIDS
  African Americans, 10, 103
  Hispanics, 103

IDEA. *See* PL 99-457, Individuals with Disabilities Education Act (IDEA)
/iECHO/I, National Black Association for Speech, Language and Hearing (NBASLH) publication, 43, 45
Individualized education plan (IEP), 52
Individualized family service plan (IFSP), 53
Institute on Teaching Cultural Diversity, American Speech-Language-Hearing Association (ASHA), vii
Iranians, cleft palate, 99

Lingua francas, European trade languages, 69
Low birth weight, 8-10, 103

Meningitis, and hearing impairment, 105
Mental retardation, 103. *See also* Down syndrome
Mexican American, cerebrovascular disease, 106
Mexican Americans. *See also* Hispanics; Spanish-speaking
   childrearing practices, 91-92
   National Examinations in Speech-Language Pathology and Audiology (NESPA), 22
Multicultural. *See also* People of color
communication disorders, 95-107. *See also* Communication disorders
   hearing/speech facility relevancy, 83
   sensitivity to minorities, American Speech-Language-Hearing Association (ASHA), 82-83. *See also* American Speech-Language-Hearing Association (ASHA)
   special education placement, 80
   speech-language pathology (SLP) guidelines, 77
   underutilization, 106
Multicultural Affairs Office, American Speech-Language-Hearing Association (ASHA), x, 23
Multicultural challenges, minorities' increase, 7-8
*Multicultural Professional Education Program—Administered Audit,* vii

National Black Association for Speech, Language and Hearing (NBASLH). *See also* African Americans
   and American Speech-Language-Hearing Association (ASHA), 44
   establishment, 43
   founding, 42
   /iECHO/I, 43, 45
   National Examinations in Speech-Language Pathology and Audiology (NESPA) Review Course, 45-46
   origins, 31-32
   purposes, 44-45
National Coalition of Hispanic Health and Human Services Organizations, 49
National Examinations in Speech-Language Pathology and Audiology (NESPA), 22-23
   geographical scope, 46
   Review Course, National Black Association for Speech, Language and Hearing (NBASLH), 45-46
National Student Speech, Language and Hearing Association (NSSLHA), 3
Native American Caucus of the ASHA
   Clinical Fellowship Year (CFY), 46
   and clinical practice, 46-47
   founding, 46
   otitis media, 47
Native Americans. *See also* American Indians; Native American

Caucus of the ASHA
   childrearing practices, 93-94
   children, 46-47
   cleft palate, 99
   Paraprofessional training, Bureau of Indian Affairs, 110
Neurological deficits, 8

Office of Multicultural Affairs, American Speech-Language-Hearing Association (ASHA), x, 23, 82-83
Otitis media
   African Americans, 9
   American Indians, 9, 47, 103, 110
   Asian Americans, 9
   white Americans, 9
Otosclerosis, 97-98

Paraprofessional training, Bureau of Indian Affairs, 110
People of color. *See* Multicultural
PL 99-457, Individuals with Disabilities Education Act (IDEA), 53, 102
PL 94-142, the Education for All Handicapped Children Act (EHA), 51-52, 102, 104
Population shifts, 7-8
Prematurity, 8, 104
Prenatal drug exposure, 8
Presbycusis
   African Americans, 9
   white Americans, 9
Preschool, 102-104
Professional faculty, 23
Professional recruitment, 22-24
Public Law. *See* PL 94-142, the Education for All Handicapped Children Act (EHA), PL 99-457, Individuals with Disabilities Education Act (IDEA)
Puerto Ricans. *See also* Hispanics; Spanish-speaking
   National Examinations in Speech-Language Pathology and Audiology (NESPA), 22
   stroke incidence, 106

Respiratory difficulties, 8
Rubella, 104

School-age, 104-105
Service delivery preferences, 13-14
Sickle cell anemia, 9, 107
SLP. *See* Speech-language pathology (SLP)
Socioeconomics
   at-risk births, 8-9
   and clinical practice, 12
Sociolinguistics
   Certificate of Clinical Competence (CCC), 34-35
   dialects, 65-66
Spanish-speaking. *See also* Hispanic Caucus of the ASHA; Hispanics; Mexican Americans; Puerto Ricans
   Central America, 11
   Puerto Rico, 11
   test norms, 11, 105
Spanish speaking, children, 77, 78
Speech/hearing facility relevancy, 83
Speech-language pathology (SLP)
   African American, 112
   American Indians, 109-110
   Asian Americans, 111-112
   counseling, multicultural, 81-94
   and English as a Second Language, 105, 113
   European Americans, 114-115
   multicultural professionals, 17-29
   Peruvian, 113
   professional barriers, 20-24
   students of color, 18-20
Standard American English
   Africanisms, 70
   bidialectualism, 72
Stereotype countermeasures, 85-86
Stroke incidence, 106
Stuttering, 100-101

Testing
   ecological validity dilemma, 14

Testing (continued)
    multicultural norm establishment,
        10-12, 104-105

U.S. Office of Civil Rights Surveys of
    Elementary and Secondary
    Schools, 78

White Americans. *See also* Caucasians
    deafness, 104
    National Examinations in Speech-
        Language Pathology and
        Audiology (NESPA), 22
    otitis media, 9
    presbycusis, 9